D0439879

Time-Limited Psychotherapy

This volume is published as part of a
long-standing cooperative program between Harvard University Press
and the Commonwealth Fund,
a philanthropic foundation,
to encourage the publication of significant scholarly books
in medicine and health.

Stephanie a. Heil

Time-Limited Psychotherapy *James Mann, M. D.*

A Commonwealth Fund Book
Harvard University Press
Cambridge, Massachusetts, and
London, England

© Copyright 1973 by the President and Fellows of Harvard College

All rights reserved

10

Library of Congress Catalog Card Number 72-96631

ISBN 0-674-89190-2 (cloth)

ISBN 0-674-89191-0 (paper)

Printed in the United States of America

To Ida
wife and mother who has always had time for all of us

Contents

Preface

In the spring of 1964, the Chairman of the Division of Psychiatry of the Boston University of School of Medicine and Medical Center, the Director of the Psychiatry Clinic of the Division of Psychiatry, and I, as Director of Resident Education, met in order to find some solution to a very familiar problem. The waiting list for treatment in our psychiatry clinic was becoming longer as demands for service continued in an uninterrupted stream, and, as is usually the case, it was not at all possible to increase the numbers of treatment personnel already working in the clinic. There was another side to the problem and this, too, a familiar one. A large number of the clinic patients were in long-term psychotherapy, so that slowly but surely the lists of therapists became increasingly closed to new patients. Some years before this same problem had been temporarily relieved by creating an evening clinic, in which chronic, ambulatory schizophrenic patients on long-term drug treatment and other patients for whom treatment consisted primarily in the administration of drugs could be seen briefly for assessment of their drug status and given, at the same time, the support that comes from having regular visits.

We knew that the only possible solution would be one that effected some change in the numbers of patients that each therapist could treat. However long the list of patients in long-term psychotherapy on the roster of each therapist, the numbers so treated remained sharply limited as compared to the numbers seeking treatment. The long-term psychotherapy lists included four categories of patients: (1) Those for whom such treatment was both indicated and being well conducted. (2) Those for whom long-term treatment was questionably the best prescription and with whom treatment appeared to wander along year after year. (3) Patients in long-term treatment who had made themselves so dependent on their relationship with their therapist as to forestall any possibility for a foreseeable termination. (4) That group of patients who had been transferred from one resident psychiatrist to another, from one medical student to another as their respective assignments to the clinic had come to an end and who had developed a relationship to the institution (transference to the clinic and medical center), so that they clung tenaciously and would not cooperate in any kind of separation.

It seemed evident to me that given the facilities and resources available, the only feasible solution lay in devising a short-term treatment program that would, by its very specificity, thwart the well-intentioned sabotage that would inevitably result if the duration of treatment were left open. It has long been my conviction that long-term psychotherapy with insufficiently or inaccurately defined treatment goals leads to a steady widening of and diffusion of content. This creates a growing sense of ambiguity in the mind of the therapist as to what he is about, and, while it may affect the patient similarly, it surely increases the patient's dependence on the therapist. The result is that patient and therapist come to need each other, so that bringing the case to a conclusion seems impossible. Since treatment is the responsibility of the therapist, the problem of excessively long treatment lies in the domain of the therapist and not the patient. Further, it has been my position that the constant exposure to large doses of severe psychopathology that is a rather natural consequence of training programs in psychiatry tends to diminish the young therapist's peripheral vision, so to speak, so that he is unable to appreciate the assets of the patient before him. He tends to develop very little confidence in his patient's ability, capacity, and motivation to help himself. It is a short step then to being convinced that no patient can long survive without his close and indefinitely prolonged attention.

I proposed, therefore, that we institute a program in which the prescription for each patient coming to the clinic would be time-limited psychotherapy except in instances in which clear indications could be elaborated for long-term psychotherapy and in instances in which therapy other than psychotherapy was indicated. I proposed further that the time-limited psychotherapy to be offered would be limited to a total of twelve treatment hours and that the distribution of visits and the duration of visits would be matched in accord with our best judgment of the patient's needs but would not exceed twelve hours in any case.

This treatment plan was set forth as an administrative decision which would be implemented at the start of the new resident training year in July of 1964. Administrative decisions of this kind will in themselves arouse intense resistance. When the decision involves undoing some of the hoary traditions and comfortably established practices of the treatment personnel, then one can expect even more perturbation. And if, in addition, the new method points immediately to the need for establishing in each case a focused issue very quickly and a mental set for termination just as quickly, then a turbulence of reactions and emotions comes as no surprise.

I am aware that the question of time has long occupied a particular portion of my interest in my work with analytic patients. It began with the sense that the psychoanalyst should conduct the analysis and his relationship with the patient in such a way as to minimize to the utmost the feeling of dependence on him by the patient. There is enough of this need in the unconscious of the patient which he brings to the analysis without having it further nurtured by real experience. Nurturing dependence is quite different from being a warm, human, person. Excessive dependence increases the patient's expectations and demands for more of the analyst's time in number of visits, duration of visits, and, most of all, in the permanence of the relationship. Then there came patients who gave me understanding of an intensely sharp screen memory, memory for a setting of strangely bright, piercingly intense sunlight, which I have called simply, the golden sunlight memory. Now I could begin to understand the criticism I had long felt in respect to excessively long analyses. I am skeptical about analyses that continue uninterruptedly for more than five years. There comes a point in the treatment of patients, whether in psychoanalysis or in psychotherapy, where time is no longer on the therapist's side insofar as the possibility of helping the patient to make further changes is involved, and where time serves far more the search by the patient for infantile gratification. Patients in psychoanalysis and patients in psychotherapy are not unlike in their problems and conflicts. Psychoanalysis, by the nature of the process, is more limited in the numbers of patients who can so be treated. However, all that we know about mental functioning and human behavior comes from psychoanalysis. Its lessons are equally applicable in the conduct of any kind of psychotherapy. Therefore, while the goals of psychoanalysis are considerably different from those in long-term psychotherapy, and enormously different from those in any short-form of psychotherapy, what I have learned from patients in psychoanalysis has relevance in my understanding and conduct of any kind of psychotherapy. I was intrigued to think through what in my psychoanalytic understanding could be specifically and usefully employed in a short-form of psychotherapy that would make that short-form truly therapeutic, useful, and available without becoming vaguely short or ambiguously long.

Our therapists had no *time* for more patients; patients were in long-term psychotherapy for too long a period of *time*. If it is time that is of the essence, then a time-limited psychotherapy program would be in order. However, since a time-limited program still allows for latitude in the use of time, let us then make *time* the issue by defining exactly how long the treatment will take—not twelve treatment hours more or less, but rather exactly twelve treatment hours. If, then, a number of patients were to be treated in twelve treatment interviews offered once or twice each week (in contrast to other kinds of time distribution), we would have the time variable rather firmly in hand, and we could take the opportunity to study the meaning of time in the treatment of patients in a way not done before.

It is hardly proper for a clinician to propose a bold, challenging treatment plan and then leave the performance of the task to others. I decided to treat a patient in twelve treatment meetings. Moreover, as a teaching and learning device which would serve equally the clinic residents and me and as a means of lessening resistance to this concept of treatment, I decided to conduct the treatment behind a one-way mirror with the residents observing and listening. This was set up as a seminar in September of 1964. A brief meeting was held prior to each treatment session in which we discussed the previous treatment session, and a longer meeting was held as soon as the patient had left. In this latter meeting, all could share what had transpired verbally and nonverbally and some concensus could be established as to the meaning of what had taken place between the patient and me. Prior to this seminar, I had worked out a scheme for establishing a central issue in the first interview and for constructing a treatment agreement which included telling the patient, at the start, exactly when treatment would end. In the seminar, we could study what occurred in the treatment sessions in the context of this very specific and unambiguous treatment agreement from beginning to end. By repeating this kind of seminar each year with a different kind of patient and with residents observing either behind a one-way mirror or by closed circuit television, by treating patients privately in this way, and by supervising residents all year long in their work with patients, I have been able to gain sufficient data to be able to come to an understanding of the elements involved in this treatment method. The unconscious processes have been clarified, and a clear-cut rationale formulated for the total procedure.

I have made no effort to support my clinical observations with numbers or statistics. The exposition of my treatment model is sufficiently clear and precise to allow for its testing by others in any psychiatric clinic. If it stimulates others to do it and to compose research designs to verify its validity, then my efforts in treating and in writing will have been sufficiently rewarded. Out of all such effort it is my conviction that successful treatment will be available to far more patients than hitherto possible.

I wish to extend my appreciation to all the residents in psychiatry whose cases I supervised and from whom I learned so much that I could add to my own experience. I owe special thanks to Dr. Robert Goldman, Dr. Ellen Bassuk, and Dr. Lawrence Lifson, who provided me with clinical vignettes. Dr. Minishima Maru read the manuscript and offered most helpful suggestions. I am particularly grateful to The Commonwealth Fund, which made this work possible by a grant that freed me from teaching and administrative responsibilities during the period of writing.

Part One   The Model

Only our concept of Time makes it possible for us to speak of the Day of Judgment by that name; in reality it is a summary court in perpetual session.

Franz Kafka

1 Time: Conscious and Unconscious

The link between time and reality is insoluble. We can divorce ourselves from time only by undoing reality, or from reality only by undoing the sense of time. Categorical time is measured by clocks and calendars; existential time is that which is experienced, lived in, rather than observed. "Each moment is the fruit of forty thousand years. The minute-winning days, like flies, buzz home to death, and every moment is a window on all time."[1] Thomas Wolfe is only one, and a latecomer at that, among the great writers in history whose awareness of the vicissitudes of living embraced sensitivity to the meaning of time. St. Augustine called a person's present the memory of things past and the expectations of things to come. This definition of the existential now needs no adumbration. In psychoanalysis, the genetic and adaptive viewpoints reflect these dimensions of time. A. D. Weisman points out, "The genetic version [of emotional development] is to the past what the adaptive viewpoint is to the future— the genetic viewpoint is only a way to recognize and to compare recurrent themes throughout emotional development."[2] Time and the subjective meaning of time are inseparable elements, therefore, in every life history, and all significant human behavior is forever linked with time.

Schecter, studying the development of the concept of time in a normal group of children ranging from age three to six, found that when they learned how to tell clock time, external factors became increasingly important in establishing time sense. Prior to this age,

1. Thomas Wolfe, *Look Homeward Angel* (New York: Charles Scribner's, 1952), p. 3.
2. A. D. Weisman, *The Existential Core of Psychoanalysis* (Boston: Little, Brown, 1965).

with many individual variations, to be sure, diurnal rhythm (the concept of the day as a unit of twenty-four hours) was described in terms of immediate *personal* experiences. These first included physiological functions, such as bowel movements, sleeping, and eating, and later such factors as interpersonal and play activities. Seasonal time, with its enormous and often unpredictable variations, was poorly understood in all the children studied. The conclusion of the observers was that the emergence of the concept of time in children is the result of the interaction between the child with his private experiences and his own rhythmic needs and an external world with external physical forces (light, dark, cold, and so forth) and significant adults, both of which have rhythmic patterns of their own. They postulate that a sense of past, present, and future follows a hunger-feeding-satisfaction sequence that necessitates an adequate mother-child relationship as well as physical need satisfaction.[3]

Fisher and Fisher made a study of the influence of parental figures on the perception of time. They found consistent evidence that the more their subjects unconsciously conceived the parent of the same sex or both parents as highly dominant, the more was their time sense an overevaluating one. In addition, a very suggestive finding was that the individual's unconscious concept of the parent of the same sex most determines the extent to which that relationship will influence his perception of time.[4] Thus, the emotional determinants of time sense prove to be inescapably related to the early nurturing objects. The development of a sense of reality is, of course, entirely incorporated within the same sequence of events. That the children studied related early time sense to oral and anal functions along with a nirvanalike state of bliss (sleep) is not unexpected.

We should not be surprised, then, that the later acquisition of real time sense remains loaded with the experiences and symbols and fantasies of the past. In the way that folklore so often exposes unconscious conflict and meaning, time as a limited commodity is portrayed as Father Time, with a beard and a scythe; limitless time, immortality, is invariably presented in the figure of a woman. Time always represents the reality principle, and the time to wake up is connected with father. By contrast, the attributes of the pleasure principle, the primary process and timelessness, are related to the mother. Ambivalence in respect to time is exemplified in our images of finite time as Father Time and immortality as a woman.[5]

3. D. E. Schecter, M. Symonds, and I. Bernstein, "The Development of the Concept of Time in Children," *Journal of Nervous and Mental Diseases*, 121 (1955), 301.

4. S. Fisher and R. L. Fisher, "Unconscious Conceptions of Parental Figures as a Factor Influencing Perception of Time," *Journal of Personality*, 21 (1953), 496.

5. Bertram D. Lewin, "Phobic Symptoms and Dream Interpretation," *Psychoanalytic Quarterly*, 21 (1952), 295.

The past continues its active existence in the unconscious at every point in the now of a person's life. Time and the unconscious meanings of time are the constant accompaniments of the now, and every now is an indivisible conglomerate of past, present, and future. The timeless quality of the unconscious was elaborated by Freud and the generations of analysts who have followed. Scott questioned whether the timelessness of the unconscious might be more a function of omnipotent fantasies than of the unconscious itself.[6] It may be difficult and is perhaps unnecessary to separate the two. In his "New Introductory Lectures on Psychoanalysis," Freud remarks: "There is nothing in the id that could be compared with negation; and we perceive with surprise an exception to the philosophical theorem that space and time are necessary forms of our mental acts. There is nothing in the id that corresponds to the idea of time; and there is no recognition of the passage of time, and—a thing that is most remarkable and awaits consideration in philosophical thought—no alteration in its mental processes is produced by the passage of time."[7]

The psychological meaning of time is elaborated in some detail in the beautiful paper of Marie Bonaparte on "Time and the Unconscious," published over thirty years ago.[8] She focuses on the notion of the "paradise" of childhood, which is popular, even poetical, although with small effort most people can recall the torment of smallness and the burning impatience to grow up. She describes a quality of memory which gives that childhood world a vision and a feeling of golden sunlight that is overbrilliant and unreal. She attributes this not only to the amnesia of many childhood events, but more to the actual experience of infinite time, or timelessness, in the world of childhood. It is not at all unusual to hear from patients in psychoanalysis a description of this same intense recollection, and it is always found to be related to close body contact with the mother. Two of my own analytic patients drew the sunny state of California into such a fantasy, although neither one had been born there, and another used the image of bright white wool, pressing close. The yearning for what once was remains vigorously alive.

Bonaparte observes that in adolescence, life seems to be spread out in a limitless expanse and death does not seem to exist. This concept of time opposes the remarkable intellectual and reality development characteristic of adolescence. Thus, adolescents become sorely conflicted because they know that there is limited time available for making certain life decisions, so that the characteristic ambiva-

6. W. Clifford M. Scott, "Some Psycho-dynamic Aspects of Disturbed Perception of Time," *British Journal of Medical Psychology*, 21 (1948), 111.

7. Sigmund Freud, "The Dissection of the Psychical Personality," *Complete Psychological Works* (London: Hogarth Press, 1964), XXII, 57.

8. Marie Bonaparte, "Time and the Unconscious," *International Journal of Psychoanalysis*, 21 (1940), 427.

lence at this developmental period is heightened by preoccupations with time. "We destroy time from the moment we begin to use it . . . for in living our time we die of it."[9]

Although there are no effective means for struggling against time, we do try. Bonaparte describes five situations in which the pleasure principle prevails and time can cease to exist. (1) Dreams in which we guard the illusions of childhood and defeat time by immersing ourselves in the infinite time of childhood. (2) Daydreams in which fairytale fantasies of omnipotence dominate, and reality and time are conquered. (3) The intoxication of love, which, with its remarkable idealization of the loved object, allows the lover to transcend time, to vow eternal love, and to ignore reality. (4) Intoxication from drink or drugs, which is used to minimize or erase reality and allow full reign to the pleasure principle. Bonaparte was able to point out even then that the psychotoxic drugs such as heroin and marijuana diminish or eliminate the sense of time and that the euphoria produced by these drugs arises from the escape from the constriction and passage of time. Carefully controlled experiments today on the effects of marijuana highlight the alterations in time sense as a major effect. (5) States of mystic ecstasy, which are not unlike the ecstatic states experienced by drug users and lovers. In all three, but particularly in the mystic states, subjective feelings of eternity are projected and given an objective existence, which effectively conquers time.

If one can eliminate time sense, one can also avoid the ultimate separation that time brings—death. In a period of history of heightened alienation and separation of one from the other such as exists today, drugs that slow or stop the sense of time relieve the pain of loneliness now and the future threat of total aloneness. For example, while in analysis, an unmarried man with powerful ambivalent attachments to his mother who was living in another city was invited to have Thanksgiving dinner with a couple who were his friends. All became "stoned" on marijuana before dinner. He noted that he continued to feel very warm about the total set and had a good feeling about it all. Time, however, seemed to be extremely prolonged. "It all seemed like forever. Time stretched out incredibly." He described the woman of the couple as very caring, very womanly, a good cook, and added that she "seemed like a generation out of phase." By this he meant that the dinner that she made was what his mother would make. Thus, the effect of the drug was to promote a sense of foreverness, of eternity, which is linked to the taking in of good things from the mother.

Baba Ram Dass, who as Alpert was once a colleague of Leary in the use of hallucinogens as the new religion, now achieves the same goal without the use of drugs. He quotes the Third Noble Truth of

9. Bonaparte, "Time and the Unconscious."

Buddha, saying that one must give up attachment and desire and make an end of births, deaths, suffering.

You end the whole thing that keeps you stuck.
If I'm not attached to this particular
Time-Space locus then I can free my
Awareness from my body and I can become
One with it all
I can merge with
The Divine Mother. [10]

The sense of time may serve as a major reassurance to the ego of its own existence, while the existence of past time, of memories, can also be used by the ego to create the illusion of timelessness.[11] Since the perception of time is always a confrontation with reality and its limitations, memory may be employed as a means of making every past event an occurrence of now, thereby reducing time to zero and giving new life to the sense of magical omnipotence.[12] The passage of time symbolizes the period of separation. Observation of the phases of the moon and other phenomena are based on this anxiety. "Timelessness is the fantasy in which mother and child are endlessly united. The calendar is the ultimate materialization of separation anxiety."[13] The remarkable ambivalence about time is seen in the common attributes of time as a teacher, as a healer, and as a friend.

All these situations constitute clearcut evidence for the presence of a sense of timelessness residing in the unconscious of all humans. An even more remarkable expression of it is the fact that no person *feels* himself to be growing old. In the presence of good health, we do not experience the advance of old age. We do perceive the effects of the aging process and we are aware *inwardly* of having grown older. The pursuit of timelessness, of eternity, is dramatically accented by the usual portrayals of Time as an old man with a scythe, and Death as a grinning skeleton with a scythe. We seek to avoid destruction by avoiding time.

Winnicott considers the depressive position as a normal stage in healthy infant development occurring in the weaning age, that period when the infant can begin to give things up, throw things away. Significantly, he adds that this normal depressive position depends on the development of a sense of time which is a prerequisite for the appreciation of the difference between fact and fantasy. In an individual who has achieved this normal developmental stage, future reactions to loss are grief and sadness. If there is some degree of fail-

10. Baba Ram Dass, *Remember Be Now Here* (New York: Crown Publishers, 1971), p. 38.

11. Franz S. Cohn, "Time and the Ego," *Psychoanalytic Quarterly*, 26 (1957), 168.

12. J. Meerloo, "Father Time," *Psychiatric Quarterly*, 24 (1950), 657.

13. E. Bergler and G. Roheim, "Psychology of Time Perception," *Psychoanalytic Quarterly*, 26 (1946), 190.

ure at the depressive position, loss leads to depression. Furthermore, a well-established depressive position is accompanied by introjects of personal enrichment and stabilization as well as memories of good experiences and of loved objects. These allow for sustaining loss without undue environmental support.[14]

In recent years, attention has been directed more than ever before to the dying patient; what goes on in his mind and his feelings; what goes on in the minds and feelings of family and caretakers; and how the interaction of the two sides confronted by the ultimate limitation of time allows for dying with greater or lesser degrees of dignity and serenity. Eissler was among the first to give extended study to the state of dying, and since death and time are indelibly connected in our subjective experience, his consideration of time is pertinent. While physical time is reduced to a pinpoint, the moment observed on the clock, psychological time, by contrast, expands or constricts in accordance with age, mood, and other factors such as Weisman mentions (qualitative fluctuations in reality sense, cycles of interpersonal activity, discontinuities of perception, and alternating expansion and contraction of libidinal fields).[15] For the child, the next day may be felt to be somewhere in the remote future, while in an adult, next week may be experienced as the immediate present. For the aged, there is no experience of future time except for that which can be contrived by such ego defenses as denial of an end to time.

Both Eissler and Winnicott attribute crucial impact on personality development to the development of a sense of time. There is no contradiction here, since Winnicott sees the development of time sense as a necessary ingredient in mastering the repetitive losses that must be endured in the course of living. Eissler also correctly points out that the indivisible union between reality and time sense undoes forever in the life of the person his timeless paradise, so that the appreciation of time as an explicit content brings with it the knowledge of death as an explicit content.[16]

Eissler believes "that society by its impact upon the emotional sphere, upon a person's attitude toward his body, upon the concept of death, and in many more ways, leaves a characteristic imprint upon time experience."[17] Surely the evidence for this is even more certain fifteen years after Eissler's statement. We live in a historical period when time has been shattered, or at least seems to be shattered, as it is experienced. We no longer measure profound social

14. D. W. Winnicott, "The Depressive Position in Normal Emotional Development," *British Journal of Medical Psychology*, 28 (1955), 89.

15. K. Eissler, *The Psychiatrist and the Dying Patient* (New York: International Universities Press, 1955); Weisman, *Existential Core of Psychoanalysis*, p. 90.

16. Eissler, *The Psychiatrist and the Dying Patient*, p. 266.

17. Eissler, *The Psychiatrist and the Dying Patient*, p. 282.

change in generations, but rather by the decade or less. The conquest of space and time by satellite communication and the immediate availability of visual events all over earth and even beyond this planet further fashion time experience and meaning into a steadily shrinking mold. Time seems to rush by more rapidly than we can comprehend what is happening.

All means of communication are now breathlessly rapid; all vehicles move rapidly; change occurs swiftly. The resultant sense of impermanence, instability, and unharnessed speed is reflected in a charged-up sense of time, such that the limitation of time appears to be omnipresent and equally oppressive. Time-limited psychotherapy has a particular suitability now that time is an ever present urgency for everybody all the time. We cannot help but feel that there is *less* time available for any of us to get whatever it is that we want or think that we want. As the rushing experience of time forces the end of personal time—death—even more urgently upon us, death becomes increasingly unacceptable. We ask medicine to eliminate death itself. We demand instant change as well as instant cure. We try to refuse to accept the visible effects of the passage of time. Thus, the enormous market among older people for young fashions, a vast array of cosmetics, the widespread use of plastic surgery, and the popularity of hair dyes and wigs—for men as well as for women. The social expression of futile attempts to slow up time is seen, for example, in the reissue of a Sears, Roebuck catalogue of over fifty years ago which has become a bestseller. This kind of nostalgia reflects on the deepest level the wish to return to past time, to make past time now and thereby to restore infantile omnipotence and, with it, timelessness. "In all human hearts there is a horror of time."[18]

All short forms of psychotherapy, whether their practitioners know it or not, revive the horror of time. Whatever differences there may exist among the various kinds of short forms of psychotherapy, or among their proponents, the factor common to all is the obvious and distinct limitation of *time*. However, despite the profound awareness of the influence of unconscious mental processes on both the development and present daily life of the individual patient, no attention, or at best the most casual attention, is paid to the subjective and objective meanings of time both to the patient and to the therapist.

Of all the pioneers of psychoanalysis and of psychotherapy, only Otto Rank called attention to a specific aspect of time and used it in his treatment of patients. He felt that the patient is always aware that the treatment must one day be finished, and, moreover, that in every single treatment hour the patient repeats in miniature his original "mother-fixation" and the severance of that fixation until he is finally able to master it and finish it. When Rank succeeded in over-

18. Bonaparte, "Time and the Unconscious."

coming the patient's mother-fixation through analysis of the transference, "then a definite term is fixed for the analysis within which
period the patient repeats automatically the new severance from the
mother (substitute) figure, in the form of the reproduction of his
own birth."[19] He adds in a footnote that patients choose a gestational
and hence a termination period of from seven to ten months, and
that the choice refers in fact to the patient's own birth. Insofar as
Rank believed that the trauma of birth stood at the center of all later
human development and experience, his approach was highly idio-
syncratic, and only a very small group of therapists continue to use
and promote his ideas. Moreover, his concept of time was a limited
one, albeit extremely important in respect to the difficulties and
complexities of the termination process in psychoanalysis as well as
in any psychotherapy.

The specific limitation of time as an unvarying constant from the
beginning of treatment and the train of unconscious dynamic events
that follows as a result not only serve as guidelines in treating the
patient, but also can provide a means of studying and coordinating
the meaning and effects of time, so that at least some aspect of the
horror of time is reduced or eliminated. None of the short forms of
psychotherapy has approached treatment of emotional disorders from
this stance. One of the critical problems in the humane management
of the dying patient is the denial of death by all the caretakers, professional, family, relatives and friends. One way of understanding the
failure to give time central significance in short forms of psychotherapy lies in the will to deny the horror of time by the therapists
themselves.

Since there is only a now in existential time, whatever the patient's
presenting distress, it is linked firmly to enduring events in his inner
life which extend to the remotest past and into a foreseeable future.
They are felt as *now*. All events that occurred in the past are not
necessarily important; only those that have endured over time and
are again inseparable from time. Any psychotherapy which is limited
in time brings fresh flame to the enduring presence in all persons
of the conflict between timelessness, infinite time, immortality and
the omnipotent fantasies of childhood on the one hand, and time,
finite time, reality, and death on the other hand.[20] The wishes of the
unconscious are timeless and promptly run counter to an offer of
help in which time is limited. Thus, any time-limited psychotherapy

19. Otto Rank, *The Trauma of Birth* (New York: Harcourt Brace Co., 1929).
20. In children and in young adolescents, the slow passage of time becomes
agonizing in its apparent purpose of delaying biological and psychological gratifications. "When will I be big enough to do as I please, to have a woman, to
control others"—all the adult pleasures which illuminate an illusory but glowing
future of freedom. As adults grow older, the gratifications of life are recognized
for their temporary nature, and the swift passage of time is all too real. Wishing
for the passage of time then becomes asking for old age, infirmity, and death.

addresses itself both to child time and to adult time. At the least, this gives rise to powerful conflicting reactions, responses, and most of all, conflicting expectations. The greater the ambiguity as to the duration of treatment, the greater the influence of child time on unconscious wishes and expectations. The greater the specificity of duration of treatment, the more rapidly and appropriately is child time confronted with reality and the work to be done.

In any dynamic psychotherapy, the restless guardians of time are aroused. It is unavoidable. We have tended to pay little attention to it until the issue of termination of treatment arises. At that point, all sorts of ambiguities and resistances in respect to termination are allowed to intrude by both patient and therapist. If we undertake psychotherapy of limited duration, it would be wise to begin where the patient is; namely, that as soon as he learns that the amount of time for help is limited, he is actively subject to the magical, timeless, omnipotent fantasies of childhood, and his expectations in respect to the treatment arise from them as he lives them now. It is on the basis of this meaning of a real-unreal, conscious-unconscious *now* that we move into active consideration of the treatment itself.

2 The Treatment Agreement and Treatment Guidelines

The treatment agreement in this method of time-limited psychotherapy reflects a studied, structured approach based on psychoanalytic concepts of mental functioning. It is designed to take advantage of, to utilize constructively in the service of the patient, the element of time that is in itself implicit in every kind of short-form psychotherapy and that is so steadfastly avoided in the mental lives of both patients and therapists, as well as in the psychiatric literature.

The failure to give time, that horror in all human hearts, full recognition has effectively obstructed efforts to establish a sound methodology of any short-form psychotherapy. The natural result has been a growing reliance upon eclecticism—seizing upon anything that seems to be humane as also being helpful. The next step in the progression can only be to assert that short-form psychotherapy requires only common sense, whereupon blindness and ignorance of mental functioning shall, in fact, prevail.[1]

The lack of any kind of adequate methodology in short-term therapy has been decried by Wolberg: "We apply the same tactics that we find useful in prolonged treatment, namely, relaxed listening, permitting the relationship to build up and move into zones of transference, waiting expectantly for the patient to acquire motivations for self-direction, and peeling off layers of resistance to reach

1. C. K. Aldrich, "Brief Psychotherapy: A Reappraisal of Some Theoretical Assumptions," *American Journal of Psychiatry*, 125 (1968), 5-37.

the treasures of the unconscious."[2] Despite his sharp criticism, Wolberg goes no further in outlining any kind of methodology; rather he calls upon therapists to make a series of compromises from the traditional, psychoanalytic-like position that will enable them to accept limited treatment goals, greater activity, and greater flexibility, including a readiness to be genuinely eclectic in method. Only in respect to the actual termination of treatment does he give any attention specifically to time, and even then he disposes of it so casually as to encourage the reader to pay no more attention than that. "Termination will be accepted without protest if the patient has been appraised of and has accepted the fact that he will be in therapy just as long as is deemed necessary."[3] It is not made clear who will so deem it, patient, or therapist, or both. Semrad and his colleagues show understanding of the need for methodology when they suggest that a sensitive and organized approach to a patient will make for a shorter treatment period. However, no mention is made of time or of the duration of treatment.[4]

Many clinicians have recognized and appreciated specific aspects of the problem of time but all have stopped short of seeing it as a nodal point for the construction of a methodology. Alexander, the only contributor in Wolberg's standard reference on short-term psychotherapy who makes any reference to the meaning of time, makes the point that since no patient wishes to face up to the source and nature of his conflicts (to face himself as he is), the prolongation of treatment always serves the neurosis. Therefore, he impresses his patients with the fact that they will press toward the completion of treatment as quickly as possible. Alexander remarks, "Of course, we are not magicians, but our intention is to make therapy as brief as we can." His use of the word *magician* implies that he knows what the patient's expectations and fantasies are, especially in short-term treatment, but even so he does not press for any specific use of them.[5]

In a vast experience with short-term dynamic psychotherapy, Sifneos has established a variable time limit based on symptomatic improvement. He speaks of termination as soon as the patient is symptom-free and is relating and working better.[6]

Another standard reference is *Emergency Psychotherapy and Brief*

2. L. R. Wolberg, "The Technique of Short-Term Psychotherapy," in *Short-Term Psychotherapy*, ed. L. R. Wolberg (New York: Grune and Stratton, 1965), p. 128.

3. Wolberg, "Technique of Short-Term Psychotherapy," p. 189.

4. E. V. Semrad, W. A. Binstock, and B. White, "Brief Psychotherapy," *American Journal of Psychotherapy*, 20 (1966), 576–596.

5. F. Alexander, in Wolberg, *Short-Term Psychotherapy*.

6. P. E. Sifneos, "Short-Term, Anxiety-Provoking Psychotherapy: An Emotional Problem-Solving Technique," *Seminars in Psychiatry*, I, no. 4 (November 1969).

Psychotherapy by Bellak and Small. Their definition is that brief psychotherapy "is to be accomplished in the short range of one to six therapeutic sessions of customary duration (45 to 60 minutes)."[7] In practice, there appears to be some confusion, or lack of precise definition, among the terms emergency psychotherapy, crisis intervention, and brief psychotherapy. The limitation of one to six sessions appears to be more directive to the therapist than any reasoned aspect of the dynamic process of treatment. In a clinic designed to provide immediate psychiatric service, such a directive may be a realistic accommodation to pressure. Time, an immediate association to both *emergency* and *brief,* is understood and utilized only in its categorical, not in its existential, sense.

In his study of the psychotherapeutic relationship, Frank emphasizes that it is the ambiguity of the situation that assures the patient's participation as well as his willingness to be influenced. The paradigm here is "I know what is wrong with you, but you have to find out for yourself in order to be helped." He is critical in his description of the end point as indeterminate, the constant striving of the patient until he is cured without any criteria of cure to pursue, and he notes that the therapist's permissiveness increases the ambiguity and thus helps to deprive the patient of a target. Frank also maintains that there is "some evidence that the speed of the patient's improvement may be influenced by his understanding of how long treatment will last," and that "there is some experimental evidence that patients respond more promptly when they know in advance that therapy is time-limited."[8]

One will immediately note that there is the least possible amount of ambiguity in the treatment setting described herein, and that time, the most significant element, will be quite deliberately employed to achieve certain ends that will be of use to the patient. What Frank omits, as do so many others, are two critical reasons that contribute to ambiguity in psychotherapy. One is that the problem of time with its meaning of separation, loss, and death is as vital in the emotional life of the therapist as it is in that of the patient; the other, which follows from the first, is manifest in the remarkable uncertainty of therapists that they can be of help in a short period of time.

The study by Meyer and his coworkers comes very close to the target but then veers sharply away. Their patients were informed verbally and in writing prior to the first therapeutic interview that treatment would be limited to ten weekly visits. The aim of the study, however, was only to compare the characteristics of patients who finished the ten sessions with those who dropped out. The

7. L. Bellak and L. Small, *Emergency Psychotherapy and Brief Psychotherapy* (New York: Grune and Stratton, 1965).

8. J. Frank, "The Dynamics of the Psychotherapeutic Relationship," *Psychiatry*, 22 (1959), 17.

therapists involved were free to manage their patients as they might in any psychotherapeutic situation "except for whatever constraints or pressures they felt as a result of the time-limited situation."[9] Fleck, discussing the study, remarks on the possibility of the ten-session dictum carrying the impact of a prescription, akin to dosage and number of pills, in contrast to the usual open-ended treatment, and that this might account for the surprisingly high percent of lowest socioeconomic groups finishing the ten sessions.

The specific limitation of time is constant in each case and includes a total of twelve treatment sessions. The choice of twelve treatment sessions was made somewhat arbitrarily. Perhaps ten or fourteen would have sufficed equally well. Long experience in psychotherapy suggested that twelve sessions might be adequate for the therapist to accomplish some amount of work with the patient. More important, to study the meaning of time in short-form psychotherapy, some arbitrary choice had to be made so that one could begin. By placing all patients within the same procedural framework, it is possible to assess the process and outcome with some degree of consistency and reliability. One can examine the work of a single therapist as well as compare several therapists. The relative uniformity of the scheme makes more evident the sequence of dynamic events present and facilitates comparison with those occurring in other patients.

There is also much to support a treatment plan which allows all participating therapists to direct their attention to the same thing—that is, to the relationship between individual problems and circumstances on the one hand, and to a rather constant operational medium on the other. The interaction can be more readily studied. The elaboration of goals and the selection of patients for such treatment may also be better clarified. Experience has demonstrated that twelve treatment sessions is probably the minimal time required for a series of dynamic events to develop, flourish, and be available for discussion, examination, and resolution. Other psychotherapists and investigators of the psychotherapeutic process can repeat and test, as far as testing and replication are possible in this field, by adopting this method.

Certain procedures and decisions naturally precede the formal treatment negotiations. First, there is the usual intake or consultative interview. This may be extended to two or more meetings in order to clarify what it is that the patient is seeking. From the data obtained, a formulation of the central conflict productive of the present manifestations of distress can be made. The formulation of the central conflict may or may not coincide with the patient's conscious motive for seeking help. The patient is generally very much

9. E. Meyer, et al., "Contractually Time-Limited Psychotherapy in an Out-Patient Psychosomatic Clinic," *American Journal of Psychiatry*, 124 (1967, suppl.), 4.

aware of the pain that he is suffering, and he usually finds some reason or reasons to account for it. But we need not necessarily accept his reasons for the distress as the most significant. In fact, his reasons may have very little to do with the actual state of mind. For example, the patient may be anxious, depressed, and in a state of exacerbated conflict with a spouse. The patient may present some fairly succinct ideas about the relationship with the spouse and suggest that it is in that relationship that the present symptoms found their origin. We may agree that his temporal connection is correct; we may agree that the troubled relationship between patient and spouse is a precipitating cause. However, we may also conclude that the present disturbance is more directly related to an unresolved grief reaction in respect to a significant earlier figure.

From the historical data obtained, we seek to relate the present central issue to significant past sources, which enables us to sort out further unconscious determinants of the present focal conflict in the course of treatment without becoming lost in an unmanageable mass of material. Further, we assess the patient's general psychological state and make a tentative diagnosis. The next step is to determine how to distribute the twelve treatment interviews according to our best estimate of the patient's needs. A chronic schizophrenic patient who is functioning at a marginal level, but functioning, may be helped over some current difficulty by weekly half-hour visits over a period of twenty-four weeks, in one instance, for example, by weekly fifteen minute visits for forty-eight weeks. As one might expect, the majority of patients in time-limited psychotherapy are seen for forty-five to sixty minutes once each week for twelve weeks. The twelve may be referred to as twelve treatment hours if it is intended that the patient will be seen for sixty minutes in each interview; but if the therapist can allow only forty-five or fifty minutes for each meeting, sessions, interviews or meetings is preferable. This may appear to be an obsessional adherence to literalness. However, when the meaning of time is to be the lever that motivates and moves the patient, there is a sufficient mix of fantasy and reality without making for an unnecessary additional complication by calling a less than sixty minute meeting an hour.

The data described here are derived primarily from my own work with patients and supported by material obtained in supervising a number of psychiatric residents in their treatment of a large number of patients. Most of these patients were seen for forty-five or fifty minutes once each week. In some instances, the twelve meetings were completed in seven or eight weeks by seeing the patient more than once each week, a procedure required when patients or therapists themselves had only a limited amount of time in the geographic area.

With these decisions made, the patient is told by the therapist that after due consideration of the available data, it would appear that the patient's central difficulty is of a particular nature, and he tells the patient what, in his opinion, it is. In so doing, the therapist has informed the patient not only of his diagnosis, but also of the goal of the mutual work to be undertaken.

Implicit in the selection of a patient for time-limited psychotherapy is the assumption, based on the evaluation interview(s), that the patient is neither in a state of acute decompensation (acute psychotic reaction) nor so profoundly depressed as to be unable to engage in the work of psychotherapy. The substance of the work here is derived from the treatment of patients who, although they have had severe and disabling complaints in many instances, were nevertheless possessed of sufficient ego strength to be able to negotiate a treatment agreement and to tolerate a treatment schedule.

How does one go about choosing what seems to be the central genetically and adaptively important issue? A clear understanding of psychoanalytic concepts of unconscious determinants of thoughts, feelings, and actions and their relation to maturational phases of personality development as well as to the elaboration of structural elements (id, superego, and ego) is requisite for an appreciation of the modes of expression of intra-psychic conflict. In general, the central issue is apt to be of immediate use to the patient if it is couched in terms of feelings or in terms of maladaptive function. Such a selection tends often to make for a broad statement of the patient's central difficulty. While this may seem ambiguous and non-specific at the start, there will ensue a rapidly growing clarification and specification of the central issue for both patient and therapist.

The most effective means for involving the patient in the treatment process lies in selecting a central issue that is both genetically and adaptively relevant, hence one that has been recurrent over time. A close study of the patient's history will disclose some thin red line that began in the past and remains active in the present, one that denotes both genesis and adaptive effort dictated by the genesis. But adaptation always implies defense. That is to say that the patient has devised methods for mastering early difficulties. An important part of such mastery is the erection of psychological defenses which will keep out of awareness the origins of the problem as well as the pain suffered at that time.

In practice, therefore, it may seem important to decide whether to pose the central issue in terms of its genetic sources or its adaptive expression. In either instance, we may fully expect that the patient will summon his characteristic defenses when he is confronted with a central issue . Understanding the nature of conflict and of defense and the significance of the latter for the maintenance of the integrity of the individual allows for a third kind of approach which will not reinforce defenses but will rather increase the patient's motivation for help. In turn, this leads to more immediate involvement in the treatment process.

The third approach lies in formulating a general statement that speaks to the therapist's understanding of the patient's present and chronically endured pain. This is the kind of pain that is recognized by the patient as a consciously acceptable part of his human condition that need not warrant denial. It is one, moreover, that carries with it some degree of feeling unjustly put upon by an insensitive world. The patient's history has highlighted this affective state. Statement of the central issue in terms of his own chronic pain immediately brings the patient closer to the therapist out of his feeling that he is in the presence of an empathic helper. The closeness that he feels effectively promotes a rapid therapeutic alliance.

The statement of the central issue in these affective terms makes unnecessary any attempt by patient, or by therapist for that matter, to intellectualize the situation or to defend himself from awareness and from closeness to the therapist. The patient cannot but help to wish to move further into this kind of promising relationship, so he responds readily to the remainder of the treatment structure and sets the predictable series of dynamic events in motion. Further, the patient will feel free to move from the general, central issue to the specific genetic and adaptive issues over the course of the next four or five meetings. The genetic and adaptive issues will continue to be elaborated in the continuing affective milieu, and the therapeutic experience, will remain throughout the twelve meetings at a high, alive, emotional level.

For example, a woman of thirty-three is single, rather alone in the city, and finds herself in something of a state of limbo despite considerable talent and substantial education in a particular field. She would like to marry, to have a family, and to engage in the meaningful career for which she had prepared herself. She has none of these. A study of her history reveals that life changed drastically for her when she was thirteen years old and her father died suddenly. One could clearly outline the effect of this loss and the adaptive efforts made to overcome its effects in the course of the next twenty years. The central issue might have been stated to her in terms of her never having gotten over the loss of her father and of her various attempts to master it leading to her present state. Although the patient presented herself in her diagnostic interviews as a smiling, rather charming, undepressed woman, the central issue was posed to her in this way: "I gather from all that you have told me that the greatest problem facing you at this time is your very deep disappointment with yourself to find yourself as you are at this time in your life." Her immediate acceptance was indicated first by a depressed silence and then by her expressed willingness to go further into it.

In the patient whose case will be presented in detail, the central

       TIME-LIMITED PSYCHOTHERAPY

issue was posed as one in which the patient was told that she "was suffering from a constant sense of nagging discontent, irritation, and irritability." She moved quickly from this acceptable generalization of pain to the adaptive efforts over time that did everything for her except to spare her from a variety of displaced painful symptoms.

The detection of the most telling feeling state and the diagnosis of some kind of maladaptive behavior are readily made in very few cases. Even as each patient comes for help, he brings with him an array of defenses which are designed precisely to keep from his awareness what he is feeling, how he is feeling, what he would wish, and what behavior is maladaptive and what he is achieving or trying to achieve with the particular behavior. There are many variations within all of the above. Some patients will know how they are feeling, but will have no conscious knowledge of the source of the feeling; others may be aware of maladaptive behavior but not recognize that they are even deeply depressed, and the like. The task of selecting the central issue must depend, therefore, on the skill of the therapist as an interviewer. This is primarily a demonstration of his familiarity with the role and manifestation of the patient's unconscious thoughts and feelings and fantasies. While free association is the method of choice for obtaining information that lies outside conscious awareness, it is hardly applicable in any kind of short-form psychotherapy. The pioneer in exploring and adapting psychoanalytic principles and techniques to a short-form psychotherapy was Felix Deutsch. In his two major works, Deutsch outlined and illustrated in extensive clinical examples his "associative anamnesis" and his sector, or goal-directed, therapy.[10] The associative anamnesis was based upon the concept of free association, but was limited in that the interviewer directed his attention to particular words, the behavior accompanying the words and the particular moment in the interview when the word and/or the behavior appeared. The words most often expressed some kind of feeling—hurt, fear, rage, disappointment, and so on. His aim was to make conscious to the patient the kinds of feelings and fantasies that existed in his mind in respect to a particular symptom and that symptom alone (hence, goal-directed). Deutsch's special interest lay in the study of psychosomatic conditions, so that the relief of the particular psychosomatic symptom could be defined as the directed goal. The patient knows, of course, that he is suffering physically and is looking for relief of the same symptom that his therapist is interested in.

The principles enunciated by Deutsch in his associative anamnesis are equally applicable to arriving at a central issue in the course of an interview, although in general clinical practice we are less likely to be dealing with a clearly defined psychosomatic symptom. However,

10. F. Deutsch, *Applied Psychoanalysis* (New York: Grune and Stratton, 1949), p. 5. F. Deutsch and W. E. Murphy, *The Clinical Interview* (New York: International Universities Press, 1955), II.

his work remains an excellent guide for obtaining information about any patient's secret (even to him) feeling state or behavior, which the clinician can then relate to the patient's conscious reasons for seeking help. The relationship between the two establishes a genetic-adaptive continuity, an inclusive now that can then be stated to the patient as the central issue, the diagnosis, the mutual work of treatment.

Thus, "Your major difficulty is that you feel inadequate and chronically depressed as a result of your need to challenge and to pacify men who are important to you," is the statement of the central issue in a young woman who had lost her father in early adolescence. She had been an only child and had lived with her widowed mother. The relationship between the significant adolescent loss and her present dysfunction was established in the statement of the central issue.

A thirty-one-year-old married man was taking several university courses in an extended effort to get a college degree. His reason for seeking help was his consuming fear of failing and accompanying difficulty in studying. In his background was an alcoholic father, who one day was found hanging, a mother chronically disabled with arthritis, a one-month-old son who had been found dead in his crib five years before, a boss with whom he was very close who died very quickly of acute leukemia one year before, and an always present fear that his job will suddenly end by his being fired. The central issue for the twelve treatment sessions was expressed to him as, "Because there have been a number of sudden and very painful events in your life, things always seem uncertain, and you are excessively nervous because you do not expect anything to go along well. Things are always uncertain for you." Again, a clear relationship is established between the drastic loss of sustaining objects and the expectation that the present and future will be the same.

A twenty-two year old female student depressively stated that her chief problem was that she was "all fucked up." Sufficient anamnestic data was obtained to support the statement of the central issue as being that she wished "not to be hurt by so many people." Early in the course of treatment this was refined to "How did you come to think so little of yourself?"

Always, since the central issue is determined by the therapist, the patient should be told that if, in the course of their work, the therapist's original diagnosis is found to be incorrect, both patient and therapist will know it and will change course appropriately.

In the course of these negotiations, the therapist informs the patient that twelve treatment interviews will be made available to him to work on the central problem and that, according to the therapist's best judgment, the time would best be used, for example, in weekly forty-five minute visits. He should add that unforeseen interruptions may occur as the result of illness, bad weather, or the like, but that these will not reduce the total treatment time offered

TIME-LIMITED PSYCHOTHERAPY

the patient. Finally, the time for each appointment is given as well as the *exact* date of the last or twelfth meeting. I consult my calendar overtly, so that the patient is witness to its role in setting the exact date of the final interview. This practice was initiated on the assumption that patients would defend themselves even more vigorously from continuing awareness of the reality of time coming to an end unless confronted with real time, the calendar. This is in accord with the observation of Bergler and Roheim that "The calendar is an ultimate materialization of separation anxiety."[11] The use of the calendar in establishing the treatment agreement serves as a stimulus and as a reinforcement to unconscious fantasies and defenses in respect to the meaning of time. Generally, the session with the patient at which these negotiations are transacted is considered the first of the twelve, unless treatment negotiations have consumed all of the appointment time.

Lastly, the patient is asked for his agreement to all of the items in the treatment proposal. It is unusual for a patient to refuse this carefully ordered plan, and why this is so will be clarified later. Patients often ask whether anything can really be done for them in so short a time, which is certainly a reasonable query. The response of the therapist is determined by his understanding that the question emerges from at least three sources—unconscious yearning for child time, which is linked to eternity; adult, realistic perception of limited calendar time; and the enormously accelerated time of the present historical period, which contributes substantially to the patient's concern about the swift passage of time, that so little of it is for him. The appropriate response to the patient's question, therefore, is a quiet and genuinely confident "yes."

It is an appropriate response because, more than anything else, it pays tribute to that quantum of adult self-esteem, however diminished it may be, which demands some degree of self-satisfying performance or work of oneself. It is appropriate also because it responds affirmatively to the unconscious demand for the satisfaction of infantile fantasies. The patient sitting before us always speaks in a "multitude of tongues," and we are well advised to know as much as we can of these multi-level messages as we formulate our responses.

The following dialogue ensued when a patient was offered a typical treatment agreement:

Pt.: Suppose I talk myself into feeling better?
Dr.: Should that happen, it would be useful to you if you would let me know that. (*The response suggests to the patient that it is his responsibility to be of help to himself by telling the doctor about it.*)

11. E. Bergler and G. Roheim, "Psychology of Time Perception," *Psychoanalytic Quarterly*, 15 (1949), 190–206.

Pt.: Suppose I feel better at the end—will it last?

Dr.: This is typical of your fear of failure in advance and your preparation for it. You would like a gilt-edge guarantee, and I can't give that to you. (*This response was determined by material gained in the anamnesis, including his reasons for seeking help. Having been given responsibility for himself in the answer to his first question, he promptly poses another demand which is not granted. Again I direct my answer to the adult in the patient.*)

Pt.: Why the short amount of time you are giving me?

Dr.: Because that's all you need. (*This response incorporates the earlier questions that center around his self-esteem as well as the patient's conscious and unconscious expectations of the treatment. The unconscious fantasy is that he will have an eternity to fulfill his infantile demands for gratification by virtue of the doctor's omnipotence which he hears in the doctor's confident remark that the work can be done in the short time prescribed.* The resistance and the demand implied in the question as well as other lurking doubts will be effectively managed by a positive response. These are the details of the treatment guidelines.

The therapist has asked the patient for his agreement to the treatment plan. The patient has his reasons for not objecting. That these reasons are chiefly unconscious does not alter his verbal acceptance of responsibility in the process. We know that in any case in which a therapist offers his help, unconscious fantasies about the outcome may have little or nothing to do with the realities of the treatment agreement. The patient is consciously free to say no and refuse to continue under such terms. Unconsciously he is far from free, but, as noted, this condition obtains regardless of the therapist's stance. It is the therapist's obligation to give the patient the clear opportunity to question and to accept or refuse.

A treatment agreement of some kind is consummated in every instance in which patient and therapist arrange to provide help for the patient. Appointment hours, appointment dates, fees, and some statement as to the nature of the patient's problems are usually settled. With rare exceptions is any time limit established, but for those cases in which the therapist or patient have a limited stay on the service, in the clinic, or in the geographic area. Since so much of psychiatry clinic service is provided by psychiatric residents, medical students, student social workers, and so forth, the duration of treatment is most often determined simply by the duration of the professionals' commitment to the particular service. Even in those cases where the treatment agreement includes a time limit, the duration of treatment remains more or less ambiguous, since a degree of uncertainty is invariably communicated directly or indirectly by the therapist. The most usual situation is one in which a certain number of meetings is offered with a "we shall see then" proviso.

The treatment agreement described here aims at making use of the patient's conscious and unconscious anticipations in coming to a psychotherapist, anticipations that become even more florid if the therapist is a physician. Out of the welter of ideas, feelings, symptoms, and incidents presented by the patient, the therapist extracts what he judges to be the central issue and asserts the time-honored role of the physician in telling the patient what it is that ails him.[12] Further, the patient knows that the stated central issue is, in effect, both the diagnosis and the mutual work of the treatment. The therapist then *prescribes* an *exact* amount of time, the model presented here being one hour each week for twelve weeks, and with calendar in hand he announces the date of the final interview. The patient is encouraged to review and discuss the proposed agreement and to accept or reject it. The therapist deliberately tones down (but not out) the patient's expectations of omnipotence by adding that if it becomes evident to both that the chosen central issue is erroneous, they will be free to leave it and to move on to the more appropriate issue.

Ambiguity in this kind of treatment agreement is minimal. If these guidelines are followed, the failure of a patient to consent will be a rare occasion indeed. As a by-product, of course, the breakage rate, which is usually inordinately high in most clinics, will be drastically reduced. Therapists often tend to underestimate how great are the resources of most people for doing for themselves when given a modest amount of help.

12. The same role is assumed by social workers, psychologists, and others as therapists. However, they have a little less going for them in terms of the patient's expectations because of the centuries-long designated role of physicians as preservers of life as well as life savers.

3 Some Basic Universal Conflict Situations

Considering the central role of the strict time limitation and the meaning of time as it becomes intensely highlighted in this kind of treatment framework, it should not be too surprising to find that a small series of clearly delineated and defined basic human conflicts emerge quite apart from, yet closely related to, whatever the central issue or focus of the treatment interviews may be.

The suggestion has been made that this kind of time-limited psychotherapy might be thought of in terms of the development and resolution of a model neurosis.[1] Although this model incorporates all the important psychoanalytic concepts central in the dynamic understanding and treatment of a neurosis, the recurring life crisis of separation-individuation is the substantive base upon which the treatment rests. Many investigators have emphasized the fact of repeated separation crises throughout life and the crucial impact of earliest separation crises on the manner in which later, similar crises are managed. Mahler's work is outstanding in this connection. Winnicott's formulation of the depressive position, a normal and necessary developmental process occurring during the weaning stage, is intimately related to the development of a sense of time and is in toto a critical determinant in respect to the later appearance of sadness and grief or depression in the face of loss. While certain recurrent and distinct kinds of losses have been described as fairly

1. I owe this suggestion and an elaboration of it to Mrs. Paula Bram, a graduate student in psychiatry at the Medical College of Pennsylvania (formerly the Woman's Medical College of Pennsylvania), to whom I am very grateful.

universal in the life process from birth to death (weaning, oedipal, puberty, college or work, marriage, birth of children, menopause, old age, and so forth), it is likely that there are also an almost limitless number of experiences throughout life that revive over and over again the experience of loss and the anxiety related to the separation-individuation crisis. Loss of money, loss of power, loss of job, loss of other prized material possessions, loss of self-esteem, and many more of even more subtle nature would seem to be a rather constant accompaniment of the life process. Of course, total mastery of this basic anxiety remains beyond mortal reach. All human beings remain susceptible throughout life. In this kind of time-limited psychotherapy, mastery of separation anxiety becomes the model for the mastery of other neurotic anxieties, albeit in a somewhat derived manner.

Failures in mastery of this basic anxiety must influence both the future course in life of the individual as well as the adaptive means he employs, more or less successfully. As a result, although expression of the basic conflicts may vary according to the social, economic, and cultural background of the patient, the conflicts remain the same for any and all patients. The basic universal conflict situations are:

(1) Independence versus dependence
(2) Activity versus passivity
(3) Adequate self-esteem versus diminished or loss of self-esteem
(4) Unresolved or delayed grief

The separation-individuation phase includes the maturational and developmental processes occurring during the period from about age three months through the third year of life. It is during this phase that the child differentiates his internal representation of himself from that of his mother. The relatively successful differentiation of self from love object is accompanied by a reasonably well developed sense of reality. The separation-individuation phase directly determines the course of ego development. The interrelationship among separation-individuation, development of reality sense, and the course of ego development will determine the adequacy of the adaptive modes that emerge as a means of managing relationships with others.

I have already noted that separation anxiety continues into adult life to some degree. The painful affect of anxiety is repeated countless times in countless places. Reasons for the induction of separation anxiety may have some or no relation at all to the particular reality situation. Nevertheless, a situation may trigger the revival of ancient anxiety, in which predominates the tortured, ambivalent feelings directed toward the loved object. The hallmark of separation anxiety lies in the ambivalence experienced originally in the mother-child relationship, and it is the nature of that early relationship which intrudes upon and invades other situations that have the meaning of separation for the individual. So it is that unreality readily contaminates many situations, so that inappropriate feelings, thoughts, and behavior are brought into the present when, in fact, their validity has long since lost its meaning.

Mastery of the separation-individuation crisis directly determines the extent to which will be mastered the independent-dependent and the active-passive conflicts. Similarly, the adequacy or inadequacy of the self-image is directly influenced. Naturally, the separation-individuation crisis illustrates its effect most dramatically, although not necessarily most pathologically, in the specific reaction to real loss seen in the unresolved or delayed grief reaction.

Out of the many complex developmental processes, a central unconscious statement about the self will be formulated and remain fixed for the person's lifetime. The statement is an assessment of how much this one person needs others in order to exist. The most satisfactory state is one in which the person needs others and enjoys others and prefers to engage with others, but if deprived of others, can give them up and find still others. He suffers some degree of sadness in the loss of one object, which may or may not continue until he finds another. The least satisfactory state is one in which the person feels that he is unable to exist without the constant and continuing presence of a sustaining other person. Both his identity as a person and the satisfaction of his felt existence are then dependent wholly upon another. Obviously, such a state reflects the most seriously disturbed early mother-child relationship in which the omnipotent mother-child unity is never dissolved and given up. Vulnerability to separation anxiety is greatest in such cases, and object loss can and does lead to psychotic reactions in such individuals. In such instances, the psychosis may be recognized as a desperate last attempt to overcome the engulfing sense of helplessness and nothingness in order to continue some sense of being alive. The accurate detection of such an individual in an intake or consultative interview leads to the appropriate question as to whether time-limited psychotherapy can be of help or whether it may even be deleterious.

Each of the four basic universal conflicts expresses varying degrees of the capacity to tolerate and manage effectively object loss. They are also so closely related one to the other that it does not come as a surprise when all four may be clearly detected emerging in the course of treatment. Invariably, the termination phase of treatment will disclose one of the four as dominant. In those patients in whom the termination phase of the time-limited psychotherapy is marked by the emergence of conflict about independence-dependence or activity-passivity, the intensity of the anxiety experienced will range from moderate to severe, depending on the degree of autonomous functioning achieved in the separation-individuation phase of early development. In the group of patients suffering from diminished or loss of self-esteem, one usually finds that autonomous function is impeded as the result of the meaning to the patient of a real loss (such as death of a parent during childhood or during early or middle adolescence), or of a loss that was experienced in the patient's inner world without there having been a real loss or even a threatened loss. In the fourth group, unresolved or delayed grief, the termination phase of psychotherapy brings to light the anxiety in connection to a real loss which had not been mourned at the time it happened. The failure to mourn actual loss of a person when it happened tells a good deal about the intensity of mixed feelings about the lost person as well as about the self, such that repression and denial are brought to bear so heavily as to keep out of awareness all the painful feelings and fantasies. The patient's conscious need for help, months or, more usually, years after the death of the loved one, may be precipitated by deliberate recollections of the lost one or, much more likely, by a spontaneous occurrence in the current life of the patient, such as the loss by death of a spouse, child, friend, or other relative, or the intriguing kind of anniversary reaction in which the patient reaches the same age as that of the loved one when he died. Just as frequently, one will see in this group the earlier, unmourned loss brought to light by any kind of current conflict situation in which the patient comes to feel threatened by loss, rather than experience a real loss.

In effect, the four universal conflict situations express all the ways that humans experience loss. The effects of loss are multiple in personality development but may be conceptualized operationally as consisting in feelings and ideas about the self that sabotage more gratifying functioning of the self. It is as though each individual feels that he needed something more of the sustaining object when he was deprived of that object. If only he were able to go back in time to renew negotiations with that object so that he could gain what he had not previously. On reflection, one may understand more clearly now why so often only a modest degree of help may readily summon resources present but unused to achieve further satisfying autonomy.

The conflicts of independence-dependence and of activity-passivity, very closely related in so many ways, may be separated on the basis of the nature of what is the regressive pull in the patient or what the patient fears is regressive and seeks to avoid. To what extent and in what ways are the patient's present wishes in the real world influenced by persistent yearning for the dependent or passive pleasures of early childhood? The corollary would be, to what extent and in what ways does the patient repudiate dependent or passive pleasures that are valid in adult life? The independence-dependence conflict relates to the degree to which one feels reasonably comfortable within oneself, reasonably self-sustaining and therefore reasonably free of undue demands on others for satisfaction; or whether one feels uncertain about one's capacity to be even reasonably self-sustaining and must make undue demands on others for satisfaction. The activity-passivity conflict relates to the degree of felt inner freedom, or lack of it, to pursue one's wishes or needs or aims with appropriate aggressiveness; or whether one chooses or feels compelled to wait for and expect others to gratify one's needs and wishes and aims.

It is evident that the levels of meaning of loss surrounding the independence-dependence conflict and the activity-passivity conflict filter through all the levels of psychosexual development. Loss of love and narcissistic supply arising out of the original mother-child relationship, loss as symbolized in castration fantasies, and loss resulting from alienation of the superego with its harsh and/or angry demands will be manifest in the thoughts, feelings, fantasies, and behavior of these patients. In all four basic conflicts, the loss of a sustaining object revives the anxiety which had its genesis in the separation-individuation period of development.

The most poignant and most distinctively human reaction occurs in the face of loss. The specific limitation of time and the framework of the treatment agreement create in this kind of treatment a clearly demarcated beginning, a distinct middle, and an unavoidable end. The beginning restores to the patient the golden glow of unity with mother, preseparation in endless time. The middle brings with it the disappointment that a relationship once wholly unambivalent will once more become ambivalent. And the end introduces the unavoidable harsh reality that what was lost must be given up. In the struggle over giving up the object once more, and this time without self-defeating anger or hatred or despair or guilt, one sees in capsule form both the adaptive means used by the patient over the years to defend against the ambivalent feelings and the basic conflict situation.

It is in the nature of this kind of time-limited psychotherapy that the only loss that can and should be dealt with is object loss. A line extends from a point of eternity in the distant past to a point that marks an end in the present. The avoidance of dealing with other varieties of loss as they come up in the treatment is, as will be seen, a means of preventing widespread regression. Each of the four basic conflict situations is a continuing effort to keep alive an impossible reality—namely, one of immortality. Among the great plagues that beset mankind, the plague of ambivalence, sparing no one, must be the first. Through it each clings to an impossible fantasy that limits or prevents satisfaction in the present. With it each promotes friction in varying degrees with sustaining objects in his adult life. The mother soil for the growth of ambivalence lies in the individuation-separation period of growth and development. The structure and rationale of this method of time-limited psychotherapy are addressed and move the patient to address himself, to the root of the plague. The treatment can diminish and ameliorate the scope and influence of the plague, but it cannot eliminate it. It is likely that nothing known to man at this time can do so.

It should not be expected nor understood, however, that all patients are alike. Each patient is unique; each has had his own very special life experiences that have been different from those of any other person and each has emerged from them with his own set of unconscious fantasies and defenses that mark him as a unique personality. In treatment we must tune in to the patient's particular wavelength so that we understand *him* as he is and not as he might be pigeonholed within a predetermined category. Close adherence to such an understanding will enable the therapist to move with the patient toward the basic universal conflicts and the feelings promoted by them on the patient's own terms—that is, in the light of the patient's own highly particularized experience. It is an experience which is shared with others only as a similar event in life. The details and the experience within the event are possessed differently by each human being.

4 The Sequence of Dynamic Events

The most significant dynamic element in the treatment agreement lies in the exact proscription of time. Philips and Johnston remark that "what is important is that the interview series has a beginning, an end and other discernible features." Their emphasis in treating children is making certain that "the treatment experience itself has a structure."[1]

A time limit is one of the elements in the structure. Malan in his admirable study of brief psychotherapy comments on this aspect of the therapy which, after all, is announced in the adjective *brief*. "The technique that we eventually developed for conveying the limitations of therapy to the patient was to put to him, at the beginning, in some such statement as the following: 'My idea is to go ahead with treatment, once a week, for a few months and see where we can get. At the end of that time we will review the situation, but if it looks as if you need more you will be transferred to a longer form of treatment. If we feel that we have got far enough, then I will stop seeing you *regularly*. This does not mean that you will necessarily stop seeing me altogether—you can ask to come back at any time for further occasional sessions if you feel you need further help.' "[2]

Philips and Johnston limited their patients to a block of ten sessions, although in some instances one or more sessions were added, as were, in other instances, a whole new series or indefinitely extended treatment. They view the time limit as only one of a number of restrictive, structuring agents and do not direct attention to the

1. E. L. Philips and M. S. H. Johnston, "Theoretical and Clinical Aspects of Short-Term Parent-Child Psychotherapy," *Psychiatry*, 17 (1954), 267.
2. D. H. Malan, *A Study of Brief Psychotherapy*, Tavistock Publications (Springfield, Ill.: Charles C. Thomas, 1963).

meaning of time. This is unfortunate, since time is probably even more an intrusive specific when one is treating a child-parent pair. In this connection, Proskauer, considerably later, picks up on the impact of time itself in the child patient by stressing the termination-separation problem.[3] Malan's treatment plan expresses a large measure of easy flexibility but promotes at the same time greater ambiguity in respect to time and misses out on the use of time as a powerful motivating force in treatment. Oberman takes very much the same position as Malan with patients diagnosed as borderline, This is more in the nature of a special instance that will be considered along with the selection of patients.[4]

It has been my practice not to compromise the time limit by making any suggestions during the course of treatment about further treatment after the twelve treatment visits have elapsed. In so doing, it has been possible to reinforce and to clarify the meaning of a beginning, a middle, and an end. A major problem in many long-term psychotherapy cases, and one which unfortunately all too often dictates that psychotherapy shall be long-term or indefinite, is the very problem of arriving at an end. Too frequently, long-term psychotherapy dribbles to an unspoken end mediated by a move to another city by the patient or therapist, rotation to another service, inconvenient appointment hours, or a chronic impasse situation between patient and therapist that relates to a transference-counter transference situation which is neither understood nor resolved. This problem prevails in many short forms of psychotherapy also. [5]

Patients coming to see a psychiatrist expect the worst. The clear definition of the central problem or focus is experienced with a sense of relief. The proscription of time touches neatly on the unconscious wish to have treatment fulfill infantile fantasies and creates paradoxically both a sense of optimistic urgency and a sense of pessimism and predetermined disappointment. The time limit is not only a proscription, it is also a prescription. The specific time limit has a message for the eternity of the infantile in the unconscious and for the reality sense and real time sense of the conscious in the adult. Hence, the impatient optimism of the child in the unconscious is tempered by

3. S. Proskauer, "Some Technical Issues in Time-Limited Psychotherapy with Children," *Journal of the American Academy of Child Psychiatry*, 8, no. 1 (January 1969).

4. Edna Oberman, "The Use of Time-Limited Relationship Therapy with Borderline Patients," *Smith College Studies in Social Work* (February 1967).

5. I do not intend to suggest that only treatment with a time limit can help a patient. Obviously this is not so. I do suggest, however, that if we understand the meaning and effect of observing a real time limit, we may not only be able to give help to a greater number of patients, but also we may be able to give more lasting and more meaningful help. Further, a real time limit promotes structure and process so effectively as to allow therapists everywhere to test the method.

its opposite, the pessimism of the adult. The contradiction between the two poses no problem for the human mind, in which contradictions exist readily side by side without influence upon each other.

At the same time, the degree and intensity of the relationship to the therapist, also limited by time, harmonizes with the patient's conflicting unconscious desire for closeness and for distance. This may be understood in terms of the opposing wishes found in every person who seeks help from another, and particularly so when it is the emotional and/or physical well-being that is at stake. The situation promptly arouses the never-ending struggle between the wish to be dependent, taken care of, relieved of responsibility, and gratified, and the wish to maintain one's sense of self, autonomy, independence, and self-esteem. The established time limit becomes and is experienced as a suitable compromise in that the patient is invited to be dependent, but not for very long.

The total effect is to reproduce very keenly the original ambivalence experienced with early important objects. If the therapist is correct in his choice of the focus of treatment, he also effects a response in the patient that is related not only to the present stress, but also to stress that is important genetically. For most patients, a crisis is generally an exacerbation of a lifelong conflict situation that may find what seems to be different avenues of discharge at different times. The treatment agreement suggests without hesitation that something can be done for the patient in the time allotted. The notion of *what* can be done undoubtedly reaches beyond the desire for relief in the present conflict state and again arouses unconscious expectations of infantile fulfillment.

Knowing the termination date at the start increases anxiety in respect to loss as well as defenses against loss. The termination date is quickly repressed, and the intensification of defenses against separation and/or loss serves to highlight much of the nature of the present central issue, its past history, and the means employed to master it. The distinct limitation of time, the selection of a focus that may be conscious (among many others that are conscious) but which is particularly cogent in the unconscious life of the patient, the confidence of the therapist that something will be done in a short period of time, and the *known* termination date all serve to fuse past objects, past fantasies, and past conflicts in a telescopic manner to the extent that the therapist becomes an intensely positive transference object very quickly. The details of the treatment agreement consolidate the various dynamic forces that are streaming in the emotional life of the patient so that a treatment set has been created which is entirely in tune with the meaning of now to the patient.

If, in this circumstance, the therapist resists every effort of the patient to divert him from the agreed area of investigation, the area of regression in the transference will remain limited. The single focus, that is, the present state around which the patient finds it impossible to act without conflict or painful anxiety in his present encounter with the world, and the constriction of time together promote a well-organized, defined, and limited regression downward through existential time, which at the same time is moderated by enormous forward pressure to the real end of time. Regression now increases in respect to the amorphous "golden sunshine" of the patient's beginnings and diminishes in respect to confrontation with a known end. Union and separation become the major poles of treatment, thereby diminishing in intensity all other phase-specific conflicts and the anxieties attached to them.

It is as a result of these dynamic events that one will regularly see rapid symptomatic improvement in the patient within the first three or four meetings. The beginning can now be understood as consisting mostly in a surge of unconscious magical expectations that long ago disappointments will now be undone and that all will be made forever well, as they should have been so long ago. The warm sustaining golden sunshine of eternal union will be restored—and in the unconscious it is restored. For the patient it is truly a literal beginning when he makes known to the therapist that his distress is greatly diminished or even entirely gone. Within the context of time-limited psychotherapy, this is one explanation of the process of the so-called transference cure.[6]

So it is that in this rapid mobilization of a positive transference, one can observe the dynamics of the transference cure within the first three or four of the twelve meetings. In essence, the ambivalence experienced and endured in relation to early significant persons is temporarily resolved in the expectation of enormous fulfillment and relief. During this positive phase, important aspects of the current problem, adaptive maneuvers, and the genetic roots of the central issue will become known to the therapist. In the midst of this positive state, the patient will be inclined to pour out much important anamnestic data and secret feelings and fantasies. The therapist will be tempted to explore one or another fascinating avenue of data, and it is in this setting that any variety of psychotherapy may become

6. Transference cures are not to be demeaned, since we know that they may sustain some patients over impressive periods of time. Psychiatrists should guard their zeal in setting as their goal the "cure" or "to cure" each patient, however. Not only is the definition of cure quite impossible, but, more important, since all adult neurotic and psychotic states are manifestations of a chronic state of dysfunction, is it not asking too much of ourselves to seek always for widespread and thoroughgoing personality change as the sole criterion for being effective? As in other branches of medicine, there is reason to be pleased with the number of five-year "cures" and even with the number of one-, two-, or three-year remissions we can effect as we employ the best means available to us. This is one aspect of the therapists' work where a self-administered reduction in therapeutic omnipotence can be of inestimable value to both patient and therapist.

excessively diffused and the goals of treatment increasingly blurred. The therapist must remain insistent in confining attention to the central issue and use only those data that relate to it. His persistence not only serves to bring to light associations directly relevant to the central issue, but also increasingly constricts the boundaries of the flowing positive transference. In this way, the tendency to regress also becomes limited, since the patient is being persuaded to direct his attention and his affect to a limited area of living.

As the therapist continues to attend only to the central issue, the patient's initial enthusiasm begins to wane. He has many things to talk about, many problems to solve, and he feels willing to do so as he continues under the influence of the beginning fantasies. The failure of the therapist to go along with him has the effect of moving the patient more and more in the direction of the original ambivalent relationship as it had been an affective fact of the patient's life, rather than as it was temporarily undone in the beginning, positive, "golden glow" phase of the treatment. Now the first glimmers of disappointment begin to appear, and these are generally heralded by a return of symptoms, or of problems, or of a sense of pessimism as to what will be achieved in treatment.

Symptoms, character traits, and life styles that have served to defend against awareness of the conflict contained in the central issue reappear or take on new strength "in vivo." At this point, six or seven of the twelve meetings are apt to have been held, and clearly the "honeymoon" is over. In fact, the middle of treatment has been reached. The characteristic feature of any middle point is that one more step, however small, signifies the point of no return. In the instance of time-limited psychotherapy, the patient must go on to a conclusion that he does not wish to confront. The confrontation that he needs to avoid and that he will actively seek to avoid is the same one he suffered earlier in his life; namely, *separation without resolution from the meaningful, ambivalently experienced person.* Time sense and reality are coconspirators in repeating an existential trauma in the patient.

So it is that by the seventh or eighth meeting, in addition to protective symptoms, character traits, and life styles, resistance will take form in lateness or absence or in generally subtle, but readily apparent manifestations of negative transference. The end phase is in progress and will encompass the final third of the twelve meetings.[7] The predetermined sense of pessimism and disappointment described

7. A beginning phase cannot be strictly limited or delineated within meetings one to four, nor the middle phase meetings five to eight, nor the end phase nine to twelve. There are variations, shading and overlapping of one with another. However, because the total amount of time available to the patient for delaying tactics is so stringently limited, the three phases are often remarkably equal.

as aroused in the phase of treatment negotiations lies in the unconscious recollection of the patient of a similar ending earlier in his life. The need to ward off and to deny the separation and end is regularly manifested in the patient's rapid repression of the termination date and/or of the number of meetings that are left to him. In most instances, the midpoint of treatment is reached and passed without any verbal expression of awareness of it. Instead, defensive reactions are set in motion. To test this hypothesis, I have made it a point in my own cases to inquire, rather blandly and almost parenthetically at about the seventh or eighth meeting, how many more meetings were left to us. The repeated response has been a hasty, "I don't know." If pressed for a further reply, each patient has given two answers— "four or five more," for example—of which one is precisely correct. If the twelve meetings have been interrupted by the therapist's absence, the patient is likely to be even more confirmed in his ignorance of the amount of time left to him.

The last three or four of the twelve meetings must deal insistently with the patient's reaction to termination. It is in this end phase that the definitive work of resolution will be done, and it will incorporate, of necessity, understanding of all the highly concentrated and intensely experienced dynamic events that have preceded it. Sadness, grief, anger, and guilt with their accompanying manifestations in fantasy and in behavior must be dealt with. The genetic source of these affects is relived in the disappointing termination and separation from the therapist in whom he has become heavily invested, and the therapist must not hesitate to examine with the patient all these feelings and fantasies and the behavior derived from them in the light of the central issue as it brought the patient for help in his present life circumstance.

The process of termination in this time-limited procedure is intensely affect-laden. More often than not it is as difficult for the therapist as it is for the patient. The dynamics of a beginning, a middle, and an end reverberate in the therapist, too. The intensity of the time-restricted relationship not only arouses doubt in the therapist's mind as to the extent to which he can be effective in helping the patient, but also exposes him to his own unconscious conflicts of exactly the same nature. That is, the therapist, too, faces the *possibility* of separation without resolution—a circumstance which one can confidently predict occurred in the past history of every therapist, in fact, in the life history of every human being. In this circumstance, resistance to termination by the therapist will not be unexpected. It is the inability to confront squarely and boldly the separation and termination process that most often accounts for the interminability of much of long-term psychotherapy. It is so often apparent, too, that even in those cases of long-term psychotherapy or of psychoanalysis where the treatment is brought to an agreed upon conclusion, the painful termination-separation phase is worked through somewhat raggedly and far from completely. It is likely that therapists of all persuasions founder to some extent at this point. The issue is emphasized here not to point an accusing finger, but rather to underline the presence of a universal problem to which therapists must pay unrelenting attention. Further, it is in the nature of this time-limited psychotherapy to aggravate and accentuate the therapist's own troubled responses to termination-separation. The number of hiding places and opportunities for procrastination and denial are simply fewer in number. It cannot be accepted as accidental that specific references to time and the meaning of time are so prominently noted by their absence in the literature on all short forms of psychotherapy.

Resistance by the therapist becomes visible not only in his avoidance of the patient's reactions to approaching termination, but also by the nature of his responses to the patient's resistance. A common experience, for example, is for the patient to inquire anxiously as to what will happen when treatment is over and he feels as upset as ever, possibly even worse. The therapist may respond in a number of ways in which the message is communicated to the patient that the twelfth hour termination will not be for real. The reply "we will see" is a frequent one and clearly informs the patient that the patient's uncertainty is shared and therefore subject to a decision that will prolong therapy.

It is absolutely incumbent upon the therapist to deal directly with the reaction to termination in all its painful aspects and affects if he expects to help the patient come to some vividly affective understanding of the now inappropriate nature of his early unconscious conflict. More than that, active and appropriate management of the termination will allow the patient to internalize the therapist as a replacement or substitute for the earlier ambivalent object. *This time the internalization will be more positive (never totally so), less anger-laden, and less guilt-laden, thereby making separation a genuine maturational event.* Since anger, rage, guilt, and their accompaniments of frustration and fear are the potent factors that prevent positive internalization and mature separation, it is these that must not be overlooked in this phase of the time-limited therapy.

Experience indicates that one cannot expect in time-limited psychotherapy the kind of full-blown expression of these that is found, or is at least possible, in long-term psychotherapy or in psychoanalysis. This can be understood as a logical consequence of treating the patient in such a way as to limit the area of regression in the transference. Because defenses are not generally weakened, and because ego defenses characteristically employed to maintain unawareness of the presenting unconscious conflict are reinstated, open expressions of anger or rage tend to be limited. However, they are present. Lateness or absence has already been noted. Irritation, annoyance, sulleness, and depression are observable. Slips of the tongue are revealing, as are details of bits of behavior outside the treatment situation. The patient's dreams may be particularly revealing of the warded-off powerful feelings of anger. Changes in the patient's attire and face may be blatant clues. Direct expression of disappointment with the course of events may take place.

The following excerpt is from the first few minutes of the tenth session with a young male patient:

Pt.: Well, it is rather a nice day out today.

Dr.: Yes. Were you at home?

Pt.: Yes, I slept a lot and ate a lot.

Dr.: It's nice to be at home.

Pt.: Especially physically. My bed at home is so much better than what I have in my apartment, and I just slept like a log.

Dr.: It smells better, too, doesn't it?

Pt.: Mmmm. I had an experience on the way over here. I was driving by school—I had to take care of a few things in my office—and getting out of my car I see this man coming down the street. Oh, oh, I've got to avoid him if I possibly can. He is an important doctor, and he is a John Birch man. He said, "I haven't seen you lately," and I said, "that's right." So he said, "What's been happening to you?" So I thought, "What's been happening to you, you jerk."—I only thought that, and I made my excuses and left. That was one guy I didn't want to see.

Dr.: The two of you go to the same church?

Pt.: Ya. He's one of those guys. Boy oh boy, get him away from me. I was afraid I might say something that was in real bad taste. He is a guy with a fine education, graduate education and all those kinds of things, but he is just completely off the deep end, just so off—

Dr.: In what way? What is your objection?

Pt.: Well, he is one of my brother's supporters, and he goes around speaking for the Birchers, and I stand for the opposite. The sort of thing the John Birch society stands for—no place for democracy. He takes the extremes to such an extreme. Anyway, he was on his way to the—clinic, so perhaps he'll get some help.

Dr.: What kind of help?

Pt.: Psychiatric help.

Dr.: Are you an advocate of psychiatric help?

Pt.: Let me ask you a question in a round about fashion.

Dr.: You want to duck it slowly?

While one might say that it is understandable that a patient might well report early in an interview some event occurring immediately before coming to see the therapist, the fact is that the patient—every patient— sorts out a limitless number of impressions, thoughts, and feelings and is impelled out of need and the pressure of the emotional situation to choose and to speak of what is of urgent concern to him. He will protect himself in characteristic modes from overt direct expression of what he is feeling. In this instance, the end of treatment nears and the patient lets it be known that he has been visiting his home where certain basic gratifications, food and shelter, are open to him. He then has to tell of his encounter with the well-educated, physician John Birch jerk who has no respect for democracy. The meaning of this in respect to the treatment situation requires no further elaboration. It is by no means an unusual or exceptional example of the kind of concealed, angry feelings present as termination approaches.

In every case, one can find ample evidence for the angry feelings precipitated anew by the termination. Termination without as much consideration of the anger as possible (and more rather than less is invariably possible) will lead to a termination that may be repetitive almost to the last detail of the separation experienced early in the life of the patient with the significant person. In this connection it may be helpful to note that in some cases the patient has been told at the conclusion of the last interview that he might at some time experience angry thoughts about me, or that he might experience a general sense of anger, unattached to any person or idea, and that this anger, too, might well belong to feelings about me. I remind him that he need not be surprised or guilty should this happen, and that he will be able to elaborate further for himself what it was about in the light of our discussions.

A summary of the twelve meetings with a patient will highlight the various issues just described and discussed.

The patient, a graduate student in his twenties, made a pleasant and engaging appearance. His presenting complaint was his conflict about leaving the parental home and moving into an apartment. His concern over this had led to increasing depression and anxiety along with difficulty in concentrating on his work. The process of separating himself from his fundamentalist, Protestant family had started as an undergraduate when he began to question their religious beliefs and had permitted himself the luxury of an occasional beer as an active manifestation of rebellion. He described his father as a weak, ineffective member of the family, which was dominated by the rigidly religious mother and by an older brother, also living at home and directly involved in religious work as his vocation. An intake diagnosis of obsessive-compulsive personality and simple adult maladjustment was made, and time-limited psychotherapy was recommended.

In the first psychotherapeutic interview, the patient's complaints and background were explored, and in this instance the patient's conscious complaint was accepted as the central issue of the twelve treatment interviews. He was told that the central issue was his conflict about leaving his family and that we would work on that, that he would be seen once a week for twelve weeks (forty-five minutes for each meeting), that treatment would be interrupted one week when I would be unable to see him, and that his treatment would end on December 18. He was asked for his agreement to the proposal, and he gave his consent readily. The remainder of the first of the twelve interviews disclosed his ambivalence toward his mother, his disappointment with his nonassertive father, and his even stronger ambivalence in respect to his brother. At the end of the interview, he remarked that he was planning to move out of his house during the coming weekend.

The accurate intake diagnosis of simple adult maladjustment made the selection of some other central issue unnecessary, since his presenting complaint was, in fact, the precipitant of his present distress. However, the additional diagnosis of obsessive-compulsive personality immediately made known to me that his conflict about leaving home was intimately bound to the particular variety of rigidities and anxieties common to this neurosis. Moreover, the family background itself practically established the diagnosis. The point is that effective use of time-limited psychotherapy would serve to refine and define for the patient a more accurate view of his problem than just the simple fact of his needing help to leave his family. It is likely that a number of supportive measures could have assured this end without subjecting the patient to a deeper study of himself. However, let us see what happened.

Most of the second interview was devoted to a discussion of his experience at a political rally. Around this subject his thoughts moved first from a neutral position about the rally to progressively derivative ideas and finally wholly personal attitudes regarding "fanatics." With this progression, his anxiety increased. He could understand political and religious fanatics, but they could not understand him. He went on to speak of his parents, the difficulties of slow and irrevocable separation from them and from his brother, their advocate. It turned out that he had not yet moved because the apartment was not ready. He now confessed his qualms about the move, about his new roommates, their girlfriends, and his envy of them. The treatment structure had already brought into perspective issues more important than the immediate one of leaving the home. Religious and political rigidity were one set of polarized conflicts about himself; the other is already hinted at in his envy of his far looser roommates.

In the third meeting, the patient had a cold which had begun with his move into the apartment, and he was overtly depressed. He wondered if he was being disloyal for leaving home. He was anxious about the behavior of his roommates with their female visitors. He felt that perhaps it would be best if he were to return to his home. I supported him in his move toward independence by discussing with him the issue of self-respect which would be at stake if he failed in his move and the pain of growing up and apart as contrasted with his yearning for the safe and more comfortable physical aspects of the parental home. At this point, it was no longer a question of discussing the pros and cons of leaving home; he had already taken action and was suffering the guilt and loss accompanying such action which is natural to a person with his kind of personality structure. Hence, an immediate supportive position was indicated.

In the fourth session, his attempt to avoid further discussion of the current problem and central issue by raising the problem of his stammering (raised more than once, although obviously never a symptom of any consequence) was thwarted, and he was encouraged to continue with our previous discussion. He spoke then of his trouble falling asleep and his remedy for this, drinking warm milk. He was having a difficult time with one of his roommates and was evidently seeking sympathy. Instead, he was told that the problem in adjusting to a new environment and the people in it were a part of life as it is, and he was encouraged to face it.

In this interview, the patient's dependent needs, graphically illustrated in his drinking of warm milk, and his search for sympathy are reflected in his wish not only to get away from the central issue, but to raise another problem altogether. Stammering is an important symptom and often worthy of deep and wide-ranging investigation. However, if we recognize that its injection at this juncture is simply another expression of his dependency conflict (stammering is derived from oral conflict), then we know that we remain on the right track by insisting that we not move from the agreed upon central issue. Rather than receiving ersatz oral gratification from sympathy and reassurance, he is moved in the direction of his wanted adult desires by being told, in effect, that such difficulties simply have to be met. The therapist conveys at the same time an attitude of confidence in the patient by the matter-of-fact manner in which he communicates a realistic fact of life.

Overt transference has appeared in the fifth interview. He opens by admiring a ring that I am wearing and then describes a good relationship he had had with a Jewish fellow to whom he had once said, "Man, you're a man." (The patient had correctly assumed that I am Jewish, and, of course, my name is Mann.) Being a man raised the question of his drinking and enjoying the pleasure-seeking aspects of university life. Typically, he revealed his automatic, psychically determined mode of thinking in extremes and the way in which his thoughts are experienced as akin to action. We discussed the case for the middle ground of moderation and how extremes of feeling often indicate the presence of opposite desires. He then described a minister who knew all the details about a pornographic book that he was criticizing.

Clearly, the therapist's response to the patient's oral, dependent demands in the fourth interview was proper. The patient quickly reacted by showing that he had found a positive transference figure; a new father-brother image, or perhaps the more positive side of his long standing ambivalence in regard to both his father and to his brother.

At the midpoint interview, the sixth, he told of his increasing assertiveness with his brother, who he feels is something of a hypocrite because he does not practice what he preaches with fundamentalist friends. The anxiety that arose out of the liberty that he had taken for himself vis á vis his thoughts and feelings about his brother had become so intense during the week between interviews that he had debated the idea of calling me. There is little doubt but that he would have called had I assumed a less firm, more maternal, and less confident attitude in relation to the patient's conflicts and wishes.

In the seventh meeting, he wondered whether the concept of a slave-mind applied to him. God was many good things, but he was not willing to accept a God who demanded obedience. This led to a confrontation in terms of facing his feelings about his brother as an evil and vengeful and destructive God. He acknowledged his long-held feeling that his brother was God. We were then able to clarify the patient's experiences and mixed feelings about his brother. These ranged from his brother as the favored one, as contrasted to himself as an obese, not too bright school boy, to his brother as his protector and hero. This led then to clarification of his brother's role as being more of a father to him than his real father. He recalled his mother and brother reciting poetry to each other and pushing father aside because "he just did not have the ammunition."

Now that the midpoint of treatment had been passed, it was evident that the ambivalence expressed about the brother related directly to the therapist as well. The state of relatively pure positive transference is very short-lived in this instance. This may be understood in the light of the fantasy, fully subscribed to and lived by, of brother-therapist as a God endowed with all the powers of great love and great hate, great good and great evil. The position that the therapist took in respect to the central issue and its genesis, and his refusal to support the infantile in the patient made certain that the patient would react to him as though he, too, were God.

As treatment neared an end, transference fantasies pressed forward. In the eighth session, he talked of expecting something big to happen to him in treatment. This was countered by a beginning realization that, in fact, nothing big was going to happen. This opened the derived areas of adequacy versus inadequacy, his ambitions versus his inner expectations, his infantile needs to be given to and his fear of needing, all creating wariness in his relations with others. Again, extremes appeared, so that he aspired to become a world famous professor while having his doubts about his capacity to do anything. I reminded him that we will be skipping a week, and he quickly added that he had other plans for that week anyway.

At the next session, the ninth, he was depressed and was having a recurrence of gastrointestinal distress. He had told his roommates that he was in treatment, and one of them remarked that twelve weeks seemed like an awfully short time, and what will happen if "you don't know about yourself after twelve weeks?" He continued that he was still waiting for the big breakthrough. He already felt somewhat abandoned, and wondered to whom he would be able to talk after treatment ends. I responded that perhaps he wouldn't need someone to talk to in the same way and he said that he tries like hell to stand on his own feet, but that he finds it very tough. I remarked that he had been working hard in treatment and undoubtedly had great expectations which now begin to fade as the end approaches. I encouraged him to examine further his feeling about giving up treatment.

He went right to the issue in the tenth meeting and confessed to anxiety about terminating. He spoke in somewhat derogatory terms about doctors who need psychiatric help, but he denied any angry feelings. He remarked on his feeling that he did not possess the "tools" to cope with life, and when I assured him that he does have the tools, he then wondered whether his "key" might open a "Pandora's box." The theme of striving was continued in derivative and ethical terms with some discussion about the morality of asserting oneself in society. This was dealt with in terms of active and passive strivings.

The patient's associations clearly mark his progression from infantile wishes for passive gratification to his concerns about his role as a man in a heterosexual world. In the same associations, he discloses ambivalence about his relations with women in his concern that his tool might release unknown dangers if inserted into a woman. This understanding of his unconscious conflicts are managed on the level of their derived attitudes in respect to his scheme of ethics and morals.

In the eleventh meeting, he began by asking me whether I had been well, a question which arose entirely from his own preoccupation, since there was nothing in the setting or in me to warrant such an inquiry. He then added that he had not been sleeping well and went on about a particular communion service that he had been to for the first time and how much he had enjoyed it. In contrast to the service he had usually attended, where the wafer is dipped in the wine, in this service everyone had sipped from the common cup. He had found more inspiration and inner strength in this particular communion. The question of my well-being was approached directly, and overt ambivalence about coming to see me emerged. He knew that he would have to leave treatment very soon but now denied any feelings of abandonment. For the first time he did not shake hands with me on leaving.

The coincidence, if such it was, of participating in a different kind of communion service with the approaching end of treatment does not go unnoticed. Facing separation, he searches for and finds a symbolic union of greater meaning and sustenance in a service in which all join together and share the one cup. The sudden break in the practice he had initiated of shaking hands with me is a good example of the kinds of changes in behavior that signal reaction to termination.

He was late for the twelfth and final meeting. He said that he had been delayed in traffic and that "this place is so inaccessible." He told of the wife of a friend who was writing a play in which he, the patient, was the main character. The play dealt with puppets and their relationship to the Great Manipulator. (He had difficulty in pronouncing the initial portion of the word "manipulator.") He played the part of a puppet who gets away. He spoke then of his respect for me, something he had never had for his father. "You make it easy. You haven't intruded yourself. I don't even know anything about you." He went on to say that he had become more perceptive in many ways and was painfully aware that he did not have any more answers than when he had started treatment. He has come to feel that he will have to proceed in an ad hoc fashion, although this is more difficult. He spoke of a book he had been reading which deals with the philosophy of living with abandon. He reminds himself not to be afraid of life, but still is. I bring his attention again to his way of seeing life in extremes—no fear at all, or being terrified. He volunteered the information that he had tried smoking cigars during the past week. (I smoke cigars and usually have one during the interviews with him.) He remarked on the similarity between terminating treatment and commencement. At commencement "some stuffy old man" gives a speech. Again he spoke of manipulation, and again he stumbled over the first syllable. This time he could make the connection with my name and added that in moving out of the world of his parents he had passed on his "strings" from them to me. Now he must find someone else. He told that in the play, the puppet breaks away and dies, being unable to exist on its own. He acknowledged that the flaw in the play was in its dealing with extremes. I agreed with him that man cannot live by himself, but that he can still be independent in ways that are important to him. The patient thought that a remark such as "Good job, old chap" might be appropriate for the occasion. I wondered aloud whether such a remark might also signify that the ship is sinking. He said that he had been asked two weeks before to consider his feelings of abandonment and that he did have such a feeling. Nevertheless, he assured me that he also had a reasonable attitude about me, too. At the end of the session, I told him that he did not have to like the situation and that he need not be overly concerned with the irrationality he had noted in himself, that along with a reasonable approach, it was important to be comfortable with the unreasonable in himself as well.

The mixed transference is clearly expressed here. I quickly came to represent both his ineffective father ("some stuffy old man") and the earlier, idealized strong father who is replaced by his older brother. Torn in his identification with these two very different men, he becomes victim to his ambivalence in all of life.

His ambivalence is intensified very quickly in the transference because of the conditions of treatment that were set up. At the same time, by rigorously maintaining the agreed focus of treatment, regression is distinctly confined to the love and fear of father-brother, the wish to be like and the fear of being like him, the wish to be given the tools of manhood and the fear of being a destructive man. As far as could be determined, he struggled with these same concerns outside the treatment situation without acting upon them in harmful ways. In the course of treatment, he reacted intellectually, emotionally, and physiologically. My efforts were directed at helping him to achieve a synthesis of insight, emotion, and reason to effect independence. In the process, he made it known that he had also internalized aspects of his therapist that represent constructive images of past important figures as well as replacements for less desirable images of those early figures. This had been made possible by reducing the intense ambivalence carried over from the past, so that separation with some degree of resolution of the ambivalence could take place. The two are indivisible—that is, the working through of the reactions to separation must lead to a lessening of ambivalence and a greater capacity to internalize an object that is experienced as good.

This patient was seen in follow-up visits three months and six months after the termination of treatment. At the three-month visit, he was composed and in good spirits. He had been free of stomach difficulties and, in fact, had gained ten pounds. He had gotten a job lecturing at a local college and was planning a trip abroad for the summer. Beyond that, his plans for himself were indefinite. He made a strong bid for further treatment when he inquired whether it might be that his stammering (still barely evident) was secondary to brain damage and required special attention. He was told that speech therapy would not add or detract from his feelings about himself as a man. He then indicated that he had begun to move more easily among women.

Six months after termination, the patient was depressed. The school year was over, and his future remained uncertain. He was resentful and said that much remained to be done to help him. He spoke of his intention to live at home again when school resumed. This was understood again as a direct effort on his part to force the reinstitution of treatment. Some of the pertinent data obtained in the course of the twelve meetings were reviewed briefly with him, so that while his appeal for help was acknowledged, he also appreciated how much of his plea for help had little relevance to his current life situation as an adult capable of making his own way and his own decisions.

One and a half years after the completion of the twelve interviews, the patient responded to a written note of inquiry about his present status. He wrote a long, thoughtful letter. He apologized for the delay in replying to my letter, explaining that he had been teaching a full load at a local college, taking a number of graduate seminars and preparing for his Ph.D. orals. He said, "I'm sure you recall the hectic, but necessary, chaos of the last few months of your graduate study, and I know you understand the reason for my delay in writing to you." This fragment makes known the continuing internalization and identification with the "man" in me. He recalled comparing termination to commencement and asked himself what had he, in fact, commenced. He had commenced his orals for his doctorate, had met and won the woman he was soon to marry, and has continued to review and reconsider much of what had been discussed during the treatment sessions. "Much of my frustration in the past is that I was always taught that ultimate solutions were attainable by faith—failure meant not God's fault, but rather lack of faith—the process is repeated and more and more accompanied by a sense of personal worthlessness." He concludes by stating that he feels that the doors of his mind are open so that he can live in more flexible terms rather than in the terms of his fundamentalist background.

Some remarks about follow-up procedures are in order. In keeping with the rationale of the treatment plan, the device of informing the patient at any point during the twelve meetings that we would like to see him at some future time, whether specific or uncertain, will effectively undo the work of the termination period. He will then feel that the end is really not the end, but just an interruption. Unconscious fantasies about reunion and fulfillment will take over once more. Accordingly, there is only one method available for follow-up, and that is for the patient to leave the twelfth meeting entirely convinced that this is the end, in fact. At any point thereafter, whether three months, six months, or a year, I have simply had the patient contacted by phone or by letter and an invitation extended and an appointment included to come in to talk to me about how things have been going. The contact is made by someone other than myself so that there will be less likelihood of a compliant response. No pretense is made that this is the ideal way of following up patients. However, it does avoid contaminating the twelve meetings, which is the important controlling element.

In the overview, therefore, one might see the first interviews as a period in which, a distinct and powerfully felt object relationship develops. During the middle phase, ambivalence is allowed to return, which then exercises pressure toward a striving for the earlier, closer, more primitive union as well as a thrust toward separation-individuation and greater autonomy. In the termination phase, mastery of separation is demanded and with that achievement goes greater sense of autonomy and a concomitant increase in self-esteem. The consequent enhancement of the ego, fortified even more by useful internalization of the therapist, serves to reduce anxiety still further. A ripple effect may be postulated in which other self-defeating concepts and defenses which exert too powerful an inhibiting effect on successful performance of any kind are diminished in intensity. The specific time limit and the central issue become the vehicle through which the critical series of dynamic events develops and is available for resolution.

Comparison shows that Alexander's "corrective emotional experience" is entirely insufficient. The core of his method lay in the consciously assumed role playing by the therapist in order to provide the patient with a new experience and a new model for identification. Success depended wholly on the astuteness of the therapist in identifying the proper role to assume as well as his skill in being something of a play actor in order to communicate a role which might well be foreign to his true nature. More particularly, there was no attempt to set up a carefully devised structure which made use of time, with its overpowering meaning, the moving force toward a specific treatment goal.

Ultimately, the omission of any kind of detailed attention to time in a host of therapies all characterized by the shortness of time is indirect but convincing evidence that these therapies simply have ignored the separation-individuation crises—perhaps because it reverberates too readily and too sharply in the continuing life experience of the practitioners of the therapies. One must recognize that patient and therapist are engaged in a mutual endeavor and that, in such a circumstance, it is the responsibility of the therapist to define and to actively bring into the treatment just what the heart of that endeavor is, so that it may be dealt with and not avoided.

5 The Therapist as Participant

There is current in this country an anti-intellectual atmosphere—
an atmosphere that is fed by the magnitude of the problems besetting
our society and by the difficulty of finding proper solutions even
for some of the problems. It should not be surprising, therefore, to
find that anti-intellectual sentiments would be especially popular in
psychiatry and its related disciplines, dealing as they do with interpersonal relations. Psychiatrists and other therapists are under great
pressure to be "human," humanistic, spontaneous, more giving, less
clinical—in fact, to give up what they know and join the human race.
In the past, moralists condemned Freud for the importance that he
placed on sex in living, and today the women's liberation movement
condemns him and holds him responsible for contributing to the
enslavement of women and for the affect barriers that exist among
us. The anti-intellectual demand at its worst is expressed in the
spurious argument that salvation lies in unrestrained gratification of
affective demands and in the enforced dissolution of all felt inhibi-
tions. These are the major goals of the so-called encounter groups,
sensitivity groups, touching groups, nude groups, and more. Each of
these groups deny reason, past history, or cause and effect and negate
the subtleties, strengths, and fragilities of psychological defenses.
Emotion, they say, is the only valid expression of one's humanness,
and so the invitation is extended to psychiatrists to join the human
race as if there were no place for reason along with emotion.

The different types of psychotherapy derive from varying theoretical and clinical considerations. Time-limited psychotherapy calls for
flexibility, activity, relatedness, and spontaneity, all disciplined by a
psychoanalytically derived conceptual model that requires that the
therapist know himself, know what he is doing, and know where the

patient is at. The therapist's satisfaction must come only from his awareness that his patient is being helped and not from the gratification of his personal emotional needs to be loved, or liked, or admired. He has no right to try out on others his own problems in repeated efforts to find answers for himself. *Primum non nocere* has an additional meaning in psychiatry, which is that the patient must be spared the therapist's problems. There is no room for license, unharnessed spontaneity, or the substitution of common sense for scientific knowledge and reasoned activity derived from it. This is no way excludes warmth, human concern, and interest in every patient as another human being, however. There is no pretense that reason and reason alone, or that science and science alone, can prevail by themselves in any kind of human relationship, personal or therapeutic.

The stereotype of the psychoanalyst as wholly passive in his work has long been with us. In caricature, he occasionally utters a throaty "uh-huh." To a considerable extent, psychiatrists engaged in long-term psychotherapy have unwittingly adopted this posture in their adherence to the stereotype and their ignorance of psychoanalytic method. Perhaps the analogy of the analyst as a blank screen, an important concept in the early development of psychoanalysis (but one which no psychoanalyst takes seriously in his work), has been retained by nonanalysts as a self-selected protective device. The fact is, of course, that most psychoanalysts are far from passive in their work. There are limits to the effectiveness of activity, even as there are limits to the effectiveness of passivity. Much of the ambiguity surrounding long-term psychotherapy results from the preconception that passivity and inactivity are appropriate stances in themselves. One can only agree with Frank that the passivity of the therapist deprives the patient of a target for the feelings that he brings to treatment and that are mobilized still further in the course of treatment. It does not follow, however, that uninhibited activity by the therapist is useful to the patient.

It is crucial to distinguish between the kind of active participation in which the therapist, consciously or unconsciously, directs the patient in the conduct of his life, and the kind in which the therapist, in addition to using his skill in deciphering the meaning of the patient's feelings, words, behavior, and conflicts, also knows how to participate in such a way as to add strength or support to assets and directions *already possessed* by the patient.

The process of time-limited psychotherapy clearly depends in good measure on the activity of the therapist. The limitation of time expressed, agreed upon, and maintained by the therapist in itself forces him into activity. Time is known by both parties, therapist and patient, to be short. It is not feasible to wait patiently for the slow elaboration of various segments of the patient's emotional life. Nor is there even enough time to allow for the development of all aspects of the central issue or focus. The selection of a focus and adherence to it are means of conserving time per se. Since these guidelines invoke a telescoping of past and present, the shortening of time suggests that the therapist can move more swiftly, too. His activity in general has for its rationale the swift-moving course of dynamic events that are underway. If the therapist fails to participate actively in the treatment, events will pass him by, ambiguity as to both process and goals will intervene, and what began as time-limited psychotherapy will become diffuse, indefinite, long-term treatment. One measure that the therapist may employ to indicate to him the extent to which he is being appropriately active in his participation is to review after each treatment interview the degree to which he succeeded in keeping attention focused on the central issue directly, or if indirectly, in dealing with data entirely relevant to the central issue even though from the patient's past.

The further participation of the therapist in time-limited psychotherapy may be considered in the light of the basic work of Bibring.[1] He describes a series of therapeutic principles and procedures which are applicable to any method of psychotherapy, independent of ideologies or theoretical systems. According to Bibring, there are five basic techniques:

(1) *Suggestion* is used in order to induce irrational beliefs in the patient. Although this may seem strange or confusing, it means only that the patient, experiencing himself as dependent in the presence of the authoritative therapist (the felt experience that is the doctor-patient relationship) is immediately predisposed to take for himself ideas, impulses, emotions, and actions of the therapist. They are irrational insofar as they arise out of the patient's unconscious magical expectations and wishes. The therapist may use the patient's readiness to do as he feels the therapist wishes him to do and stimulate the patient to make certain changes in his life.

(2) *Abreaction* makes it possible for the patient to relieve tension through the discharge of emotion. Bibring points out what continues to remain unrecognized, namely, that the discharge of emotion is of greater value in validating for the patient what it is that troubles him than in effecting any kind of quick cure, or even being a major factor in cure.

(3) *Manipulation* lends itself most easily to misunderstanding and to misuse. Neither guidance nor advice is meant. Rather, manipulation means "influence through experience." For example, the patient expects the authority to tell him what to do, but the therapist tells him that he is free to do as he pleases, or that the dependent patient must assume responsibility for himself. Manipulation includes a

1. E. Bibring, "Psychoanalysis and the Dynamic Psychotherapies," *Journal of the American Psychoanalytic Association*, 2 (1954), 745.

number of curative agents which may be subsumed under the general heading of "learning from experience." To a degree, there is some similarity between this concept and Alexander's corrective emotional experience, without the role playing of the latter. As a result of his understanding of the patient's characteristic modes of doing business with others, the therapist deliberately refuses to be the "straight man" in the exchange, but rather places the patient in a position where he may *learn* that his characteristic response is inappropriate, unnecessary, and self-defeating.

(4) *Clarification.* In all patients there is the possibility for a high degree of self-awareness if the therapist recognizes that a host of important feelings, ideas and conclusions lie scattered in the pre-conscious mind of the patient. The carefully listening therapist hears bits of important data and makes equally important observations of behavior at a number of points separated in time throughout the interview. The patient cannot keep track of them, engaged as he is in a highly emotional piece of work. The therapist does keep track, brings important bits together, and presents them to the patient as a unified concept. The patient immediately recognizes the weight and value of the clarifying statement and accepts it without resistance. The therapeutic effect consists in detachment of the ego through greater self-awareness, which brings more realistic knowledge of the self and of the environment.

(5) *Interpretation.* In sharp contrast to clarification, interpretation "aims at changes in the ego and indirectly of other functional systems of the personality that permit lifting unconscious conflicts to consciousness so that causal determinants of the various disorders are modified or removed." An interpretation properly brings to the patient's awareness that which was not known to him consciously at all. Together, clarification and interpretation are productive of insight.

Bibring notes that the method used to gain material from the patient determines the scope and quality of the produced material. Adherence to the central issue demonstrates very sharply the correctness of this statement and supports my thesis that such adherence will limit the area of regression in the transference.

In addition to the five basic techniques, Bibring adds four therapeutic processes:

(1) The production of material
(2) The utilization of material, mainly by the therapist
(3) The assimilation of this utilization by the patient
(4) The processes of reorientation and readjustment

These will also be noted as distinct constituents in the treatment process. The prolonged and repetitive testing out and learning in the reorientation and readjustment process that Bibring speaks of is accomplished in time-limited therapy in the last third of the treatment interviews.

In undertaking psychotherapy in which time is strictly limited, the therapist must begin with a sense of optimism about his ability to be of help in so short a time as well as about the patient's capacity to profit from it. Surely, optimism is a form of suggestion since it is communicated very quickly to the patient. Actually, it is a rare patient who is not silently searching the therapist's face and behavior for clues as to his optimism. One is keenly aware of this in medical and surgical patients; it is more subtle but equally powerful in psychiatric patients. In long-term psychotherapy or in psychoanalysis, there is room for the therapist to convey to the patient his uncertainty or even pessimism in negotiating the treatment agreement. Treatment may even be a trial run as agreed upon by both. There is not enough time in time-limited psychotherapy for trial runs, for a "we shall see" construction. If we begin from the premise that we can be of help to a patient, if we carefully limit our goals and our ambitions, and if we understand the treatment method that we are employing, then only one more precondition is required—the conviction that, given a modicum of help, all human beings have emotional, intellectual, and adaptive assets that they are ready to channel into reasonably gratifying directions. It is imperative that we appreciate the modesty of our treatment goals and our understanding of what a patient can do for himself. The therapist is not asked to assume a Pollyanna-like attitude; rather to communicate and suggest and induce a state of mind in the patient which will allow him to begin a task that he can in fact bring to completion. The designation *patient* does not mean that adaptive assets have disappeared. They may disappear if the therapist chooses to ignore them or forces them out of sight. The therapist's sense of optimism will flourish naturally as he understands each step of the way in its unconscious meaning to the patient.

One patient, after the treatment proposal had been fully outlined, inquired about medication. She had been rather heavily medicated on various tranquilizers, sedatives, and antianxiety drugs for a number of years by different nonpsychiatrist physicians. I asked if she thought she could abstain until our next meeting a week hence. She did not think so, fearing the undue intensity of her anxious feelings. At this point, I repeated the terms of the treatment agreement including the central issue. She suddenly asked, "Do you really think I can be helped in so short a time?" Her response to my affirmative reply was, "In that case I can stay off for a week, anyway." In fact, she took no further medication throughout her treatment.

Optimism can be differentiated from uncritical faith on the part of the therapist as to his effectiveness and, at the same time, can take studied advantage of the unconscious magical needs and wishes of the patient. In all doctor-patient relationships, patients ascribe some degree of omnipotence to their physicians. The greater the sense of confidence in the doctor (we say then that the patient has more *faith* in his doctor), the greater the expectations of the patient for relief are pinned to magical expectations of the doctor's power to heal. Some physicians, including psychiatrists, exploit this kind of blind faith by presenting themselves as all-knowing and all-powerful. If they can join such a presentation with appropriate aggressive, confident, take-charge personality styles, they can often induce rapid relief in the patient. Generally, neither doctor nor patient can account for the "cure." But the patient has no need to seek further than his faith in the doctor, and the doctor dares not explore the nature of his success lest he undo himself.

In any initial patient-doctor encounter, the skill with which the patient's anxieties are managed determines the extent to which magical expectations are enhanced. The influence of bedside manner, whether at the bedside or in the office, is universally experienced and acknowledged. In time-limited psychotherapy, optimism in the therapist is based to begin with on his understanding that the specific details of treatment to be offered the patient will, in fact, stimulate the unconscious magical expectations of the patient, and that as a result there will follow the sequence of dynamic events which he will then use toward helping the patient come to terms with the immediate *and the genetic* sources of the current central issue. Properly conducted, this kind of psychotherapy will end with the patient relying less on magical fulfillment and more on his own realistic assets and capabilities.

The activity of the therapist begins, therefore, with his active assessment of the central issue, his presentation of it to the patient, his proposal of the treatment agreement, and his optimism and conviction that he and the patient can do the work set before them successfully.

In the beginning phase, with rapid development of positive transference, the patient tends to pour out many details of his present and past experiences relating to the central issue. The activity of the therapist will tend to center around keeping the patient to the central issue, freely raising questions in order to elaborate focal data, and offering clarifications. Clarifications of present and past experience in terms of the patient's thinking, feeling, and behavior mean bringing together pieces of information that are scattered both in the mind and in the verbal account of the patient, information that is known and readily recognized by him when crystallized and brought together by the therapist. This is in contrast to interpretations, which consist in making conscious for the patient that which was entirely unconscious, entirely out of awareness, and not recognized by him as belonging to the contents of his own mind. Clarifications rarely meet with resistance, while interpretations usually do.

In this setting of high expectations in an atmosphere in which the patient feels enormously understood, it is not surprising to find that a considerable degree of abreaction may also take place. It may be in the nature of tears or of any of the feelings which are expressive of the sense of self-justification. Rather than being directed against anyone, the emerging, highly charged feelings tend to be more in the nature of sharing with the therapist the long locked up sentiments of the patient about himself. The therapist will gain much information for later use and should participate empathically in the further clarification of the data and of the feelings being expressed. The stereotype of the therapist as a nonreacting blank screen should also be laid to rest. His activity consists in responding naturally, but modestly. The patient needs his sensitive responsiveness and also his strength. Too little or no responsiveness is experienced by the patient as insensitive coldness and as the imposition of a frightening barrier to closeness. Too much responsiveness may signal to the patient uncertainty, weakness, and even failure to understand. In any case, and in every case, the patient needs a certain distance between himself and the therapist in order to maintain some sense of autonomy, of self, of differentiation from the other. This consideration, so vital to the need of every person to maintain some sense of his unique self, is too often ignored by the too active therapist and by the therapist who regards the encounter with the patient as one involving two persons entirely equal in every respect. If this were true, what then is the patient doing in coming to seek help? Some of the so-called encounter groups violate this principle of the unique self grossly and at times brutally.

Even in the beginning phase of treatment, the therapist is active in supporting, encouraging, and educating the patient. Support and encouragement are directed to those parts of the patient's feelings, thoughts, and behavior which have been devoted to the struggle for mastery in constructive or partially constructive ways. The patient may have long felt that his genuine efforts at mastery have gone unrecognized. He may be unaware of other of his efforts that are deserving of support and encouragement. Interventions of this kind by the therapist will help to increase the patient's self-esteem, which is a significant self-help tool in every case.

There is no room whatsoever for fabricated support and encouragement. It is imperative that the patient incorporate the therapist's activity with what he feels to be truth in his own life. Any other kind of support and encouragement is likely to be reminiscent of the sometimes well-intended but often misguided or rejecting efforts of the patient's relatives and friends. Moreover, he may have excellent grounds for suspecting the therapist's capacity to understand the sincerity of his effort. One must choose judiciously what it is that he will support and encourage. The need of the therapist to win the patient's good will by the bounteousness of his warmth and support will imperil the patient-therapist relationship as well as the outcome of treatment. Nor does support and encouragement mean giving guidance and advice. In a world where protests against the constantly mounting encroachments on individuality are extremely popular (and in many ways are appropriate), there are an amazing number of people in the so-called helping professions who are dedicated to the idea of telling *others* what to do and how to do.

The activity of the therapist as an educator is important in all varieties of psychotherapy or in psychoanalysis. Education may be direct and imply the transmission of information, sometimes specifically medical and more often psychological in nature.

Or education may be rather reeducation. In long-term psychotherapy, and more so in psychoanalysis, information-giving is withheld while the patient's own conceptions, misconceptions, and distortions about the particular issue are elaborated. As a result, what the patient thought and felt to be the case on the basis of his own inner perceptions is redefined by bringing inner experience into harmony with reality. This is particularly relevant in the working through of the transference.

There is still another kind of educational activity, and that is the kind of education arising out of the therapist's manipulative (Bibring) activity. This is, for the most part, experiential, involving learning through experience, the new experience being the failure of the therapist to respond as the patient expects on the basis of his own, long-held character trait or personality style.

In this method of psychotherapy, all three educational modes are employed—direct information, reeducation, and manipulation. Throughout the twelve treatment interviews, opportunities for educating the patient in all three ways will be available and should be used. The specific limitation of time may, in fact, force a certain amount of direct education by the therapist. There is not sufficient time for elaborating every misconception or distortion; nor for that matter is there enough time to do this to every last available detail, even with the central issue. The patient can be given direct information about some aspect of the history of the central issue which he can use to clarify for himself how he came to feel the way he does. The information given the patient is drawn from the patient's history and retranslated in the light of general psychoanalytic theory.

A young woman suffering depression, lack of confidence, low self-esteem, and an inability to feel acceptable to young men disclosed that a good deal of her self-recriminations lay in her conviction that she had harmed, even killed, her mother. Her mother had been stricken with cancer shortly after the patient's birth and had been in and out of hospitals many times before she died when the patient was five years old. The last time that the mother left the house for the hospital, the patient was asked to keep looking at a tank of tropical fish until told she could turn around. On signal, she turned, saw that her mother was gone, and never saw her again. To add further to her pain, she was not permitted to attend the funeral. As a point of information, she was told how any child would come to understand such a series of tragic events, and that, in her case, it was made even worse because of the unusual sequence of events that made her feel so responsible for what was happening.

The patient can be taught about sibling rivalry, masturbation, the function of fantasy, and the universality of so many kinds of wishes, daydreams, and fears. In no way is a lecture or even a semblance of a lecture suggested. Rather, a simple and direct statement of the psychological fact is made, and its connection to the central issue is clearly designated. At any point in the twelve meetings, the intensity of the relationship to the therapist will embellish the value to the patient of such "teachings."

This is especially true before the work of termination and separation has become the principal issue. Teaching is most effective when it occurs in a positive relationship and when a certain amount of idealization is present. In short, we may again take advantage of the patient's affective state and his need for gratification, but in such a way that he is helped to move closer to an appreciation of the reality in which he lived and lives, rather than to his fantasy about the same experience.

The direct communication of psychological facts may seem to some to be little more than an intellectual exercise that is interesting and useful to the therapist in a short-form psychotherapy, but probably not very useful to the patient. I have already noted the role of a positive transference that serves to make the words of the therapist (and therefore the meaning of the words) a precious commodity for the patient. Furthermore, each bit of information communicated in this way by the therapist is stimulated by data related to the central issue and is made known to the patient entirely within that context. Thus, a host of thoughts, feelings, and recollections are brought to bear more and more on one central issue. The direct inclusion of information from the therapist which is equally central to the central issue means that it is incorporated as part of an intense affective mixture, so that the purely intellectual aspect of the information is considerably diminished.

The participation of the therapist throughout the beginning phase is relatively easy. The total dynamic set of the patient favors the therapist in his work. The smoothly functioning gears begin to grind in the middle phase. Improvement in the patient tends to reach a plateau, and the first glimmers of disappointment become known either in the stated failure to improve further, a return of complaints, or, more often, a sense of withdrawal, of moving away from the therapist. The patient may have less to say or may feel that all that needed to be said has already been said. Often the patient conveys an attitude that asks, "Where do we go from here?" Clearly the patient's enthusiasm has begun to wane.

The therapist must continue undeterred in his efforts to elaborate and clarify further the central issue and should also now be on the alert for every sign of resistance. The manifestations of resistance will be found to be directly related to the patient's transference. This statement deserves emphasis, because the therapist may readily respond to the signs of relapse or growing disappointment with the feeling that he, too, has gone as far as he can. All his earlier doubts as to his ability to be of help with so little time available to him may reappear, and a troubling sense of helplessness may whisper to him that he has no more to offer to the patient. The true state of the matter is that the therapist's "magic" and carefully calculated support has moved in the mind of the patient from that which is given to the patient by the fantasied all-giving, all-loving early important person to the ambivalently perceived early person. The fact, too, is that we have no magic to offer; we can only offer our skilled assistance in a mutual task. If the therapist matches the patient's feelings of disappointment and helplessness with similar feelings in himself, the patient can move in one of two directions. He may convince the therapist that a long or longer term of treatment is an absolute necessity and thereby preserve an ambivalent, clinging, dependent relationship, which may or may not be resolved over the long haul; or he may discontinue treatment and repeat, in remarkable detail, the same kind of separation without resolution suffered earlier in his life.

However, we can be different from the early, ambivalently experienced person in very important ways. We need not respond, at this sensitive juncture in treatment, like a repetition of that past experience fully expected now by the patient. Now the patient must be given every opportunity to verbalize his ambivalent feelings. We must *clarify* resistances that are conscious in the patient and now, for the first time in the treatment regime, we begin to use the accumulated data to *interpret* the patient's reactions to us. The clarification is an acknowledgment by the therapist that the patient is justified in his feelings of disappointment and that his total reaction is understandable, since we are not doing all that he had anticipated, and we are, in truth, disappointing him. The interpretation is made in the light of the repetition with the therapist of the patient's earlier experiences with a significant person—and we have the data in hand to be able to identify the significant person without hesitation.

Thus, as the patient begins to make moves to withdraw from us, we seek to bring him closer. It is accomplished by drawing upon the resources of the patient (and they are always there) to begin to feel and to know in what ways the past has invaded a certain sector of his present life. In bringing all this into the open, into clear consciousness, we can help the patient to a position where it is not, as it has always been for him, a matter of unconsciously blaming himself or some others, but rather is a matter of best serving his own needs by coming to the realization that he has been fighting a battle with ghosts. While this is certainly a far too simplistic conception of the skein of developmental events and circumstances that leads to neurosis, it remains nevertheless a supportable statement as to the end result of the underlying unconscious process. Increasingly in treatment the patient is offered reality in an atmosphere that supports his own efforts to meet and join it.

Usually comprising the middle four of the twelve sessions, this period of treatment is marked by the plateau in improvement as reported by the patient, the growing hesitation in the flow of material, and, most of all, by the passing of the midpoint of the treatment interviews. It is usually the case that once the midpoint has been passed, the patient will begin to communicate this information. The manner of communication will depend on the personality of the patient and will be related even more directly to the presenting problem or central issue. The patient who has concealed his problem and defended himself against awareness of his problem in a particular kind of behavior may again begin to display the same behavior, albeit in an attenuated or more disguised fashion. For example, a young woman who had been promiscuous and who had recovered her self-respect in the course of the treatment to date, began another bed relationship, ostensibly on the basis of having found "the right man" at long last. The patient who presented symptoms may report the return of one or another of them. Another patient may maintain his improvement, but will talk about future plans which appear to be wholly apart and without any reference whatsoever to his therapeutic experience. Recollections of past endings, deaths, marriages, and departures may appear.

Through all these the therapist keeps close tabs on data that he will need for working through the termination phase. Simultaneously, he assesses the strength of the patient's growing ambivalence and the extent to which the patient is beginning himself to prepare for termination. These assessments become guidelines for helping the therapist to decide on the use and timing of interpretations, exposure, and discussion. Failure to make them and to act in line with them will lead to heightened resistance, which might include absences or even the breaking of treatment. The therapist may begin to make his first sallies in respect to the coming end of treatment as a way of gaining information about the patient's defenses against it. Clarification, support, education, and interpretation continue and are continuous around the central issue only.

While the end phase technically begins with the ninth interview, the varieties of human behavior are such that for some patients it begins with the sixth or seventh, with some by the tenth or eleventh, and with some there is no conscious acknowledgment of it until the very last meeting. These latter situations will occur only if the therapist has made no effort to focus attention on the fact of termination. In no case should a patient be allowed to ward off the confrontation with the end beyond the beginning of the tenth session. The therapist must reserve for himself no less than the last three meetings for the purpose of dealing directly with termination, the patient's feelings and reactions to it, and the centrality of all these reactions to the conflict that brought him to treatment.

The reaction of patients to termination in time-limited psychotherapy sharply points up the fallacy in attributing what transpires to the exclusive fact of dependence on the therapist. Granted that in any long-term psychotherapy or in psychoanalysis, dependence on the therapist is a distinct factor, nevertheless, even in those therapies it is an oversimplification to speak only of dependence and the task of undoing it. In time-limited psychotherapy, certainly the prolonged relationship which in itself lends to dependence does not exist. However, the telescoping of dynamic events stimulated by and immediately an intrinsic part of an intensely experienced existential now leads to an intense termination reaction not unlike that seen in longer therapies. What stands out vividly is the struggle around the refusal to relinquish infantile and childhood wishes in favor of the uncertain pleasures of adult reality. Adult reality means accepting the sense of the end of time, of the end of one's self. Clinging to the therapist means clinging to what was and to the fantasy that what was shall forever be—namely, eternity. Thus, dependence on the therapist has a much broader significance than is usually implied when we speak of dependent wishes with their primary meanings of being held, warmed, fed, and loved. While the sense of eternal time is attached in the unconscious to the mother, it is also independent of the mother insofar as time and space have an existence of their own, apart from people. Warmth, sustenance, and love have meaning only in relation to others.

Clinging to the therapist is, therefore, as much a means of keeping eternity alive as it is keeping alive the possible fulfillment of unfilfilled pleasures in respect to early sustaining objects. The clinging is an extremely active process which aims at maintaining intact the original ambivalent posture. Without resolution, all possibilities for gratification of all body pleasures and for the continuing sense of eternity remain open. No wonder, then, that termination is a painful and difficult process in all therapies for both patient and therapist.

It is in reference to the conflict about early body pleasures that we so call a hostile-dependent relationship. Positive feelings, love, magical expectations, and the desire to grow up and away from the important person, are always present. Also present, and serving to prevent growth and movement away, are resentment, anger, fear of retalia-tion, and an encompassing sense of guilt. These are the heart of the ambivalence that ties the patient to the past as he struggles to come to terms with the present. The end phase of the twelve treatment interviews has as its goal the undoing of the early, unresolved ambiv-alent relationship that is still exercising influence unconsciously in the present life of the patient, particularly in the major present conflict that brought the patient for help. Reality factors in the present conflict situation are but vehicles for the repetition, better, the intensification, of the earlier relationship conflict. The past and the present are always fused. Neurotic conflict can only occur in some kind of relationship struggle, certainly never in a vacuum involv-ing no one but the patient and never limited to the kind of relation-ship struggle that exists only in the present.

Herein lies the stressful situation for patient and therapist that is the termination phase. Separation must take place; the date is known, and stubborn and frightened resistance confronts the therapist. The doubts of the therapist as to his effectiveness are again readily aroused. at this point when the patient takes refuge once more in symptoms, distressing complaints, or disturbing behavior. At the same time, the therapist must confront his own ambivalence in respect to the same conflicts within himself as these are exposed by the patient.

Nevertheless, the therapist must remain insistent that the patient examine his feelings about the therapist as the end nears. Patients' responses vary. Some will hold firmly that they have no particular feelings about it. This is an extreme in which denial remains para-mount. At the other end of the spectrum is a keen awareness of resentment, regret, sadness, and gratitude. A rather common defen-sive manoeuver by the therapist is his refusal to acknowledge that he is really very important to the patient, since, after all, there has been so little time. Further, his experience with other and longer forms of therapy has demonstrated to him how long it can take for a patient to invest enough of himself in the therapist as to make the therapist of significant emotional importance to him. With this kind of ration-alization, the therapist can easily overlook the fact that the specific process he has been engaged in with the patient has made of the limitation of time a powerful instrument for the enormous invest-ment by the patient in him.

In all cases, the alert therapist will find ample evidence to interpret the reaction to separation, always in two concurrent contexts: first, the feeling that existed in relation to an earlier figure and now experienced with the therapist; second, the displacement of the same feelings and behavior for the same reasons, embellished more or less by present reality, in the conflict situation that created the need for help. The interpretations offered the patient include the past, the present, and the therapist. However, it should be emphasized, emphatically emphasized, that the interpretations are not couched in terms of libidinal and aggressive developmental fantasies, even though data for such interpretations have been provided by the patient unknowingly, but very explicitly. The unconscious feelings and fantasies from the past, their invasion into the present, and their intrusion into the relationship with the therapist are interpreted in terms of the adaptive modes of management that have emerged as the feeling and behavioral style of the patient, lived out now in exquisite detail in relationship to the therapist.

It is well to remember that in general, the patient prefers either to prolong the treatment or, failing that, to leave with his ambivalence intact. The latter can be prevented, or at least greatly minimized, by the therapist's relentless attention to and by appropriate interpretation of conscious and unconscious responses of the patient. The therapist's vigilance and persistence and courage will be rewarded by the recognition and acknowledgement by the patient of the substance of his ambivalence. A setting of warmth, support, encouragement, and strength serves well the patient's desire and need to incorporate the therapist as a good, nonambivalent object and to leave treatment with the kind of internalized object that promotes growth and the capacity to move away independently. This, after all, is the root of the acceptance of reality and constructive adaptation to it. No one arrives at a reasonable acceptance of reality by himself.

The task is difficult but it can be done. The therapist must possess a genuine understanding of the course of dynamic events that can be mediated through his efforts to a productive and creative end for the patient. It would hardly be amiss to suggest that both the understanding of the process and the performance of the task itself demands a high degree of knowledge of the self. Such self-knowledge can be attained by the therapist only through his own personal psychoanalysis. Does this mean that no therapist but the analyzed therapist can be effective in this kind of psychotherapy? It is axiomatic in medicine that the words *never* and *always* cannot be used. The sensitive, gifted, nonanalyzed therapist may do superbly with certain cases. The analyzed, sensitive, and gifted therapist will do superbly in many more cases. A personal analysis will help any therapist do better what he has been doing all along. The responsibility of all therapists is to foster in their patients that *inner* freedom which leads to maturity, acceptance of reality, and independence.

Another summary of the twelve interviews with a patient may clarify further the participation of the therapist in the therapeutic process. The patient was a graduate student nearing thirty. Out of the preliminary interview a number of related complaints emerged:

— A feeling that he has always drifted without motivation and without any feeling that any path is really open to him even if he knew what it was
— Lack of self-confidence
— Social anxiety, which he managed with alcohol, at times to great excess
— Frequent, rather typical anxiety attacks
— Anxiety at times at school, such that he was unable to eat his lunch until the day was over and he had returned to his home
— A fear of flying, which he said "limits my goals in this day and age"

He denied profound feelings of depression and never felt suicidal.

From his past history we learn that he has one older sister. He was born during World War II, while his father was in the service. His father, a successful man in his field, moved the family considerably during the patient's early school years. Entirely uncertain about his future when he graduated from high school, he was encouraged to go to a school abroad with the idea that the experience would stimulate his independence and allow him to come to terms with a future goal. He went, but left the school after several months and spent the remainder of the year in a large European city, "goofing around." There he learned about alcohol, and there, too, he had his first sexual experiences. These included an episode of gonorrhea. He returned to this country when the year was over and enrolled at a university. During the next four years, he made his way to three different universities, doing well at none of them. However, he did manage to get his bachelors degree and just made it into graduate school. At the time he was seen, he was living with a girl weekends and at home during the week. His sexual relations were pleasurable, although he was concerned about recurrent urethral burning. He had been seeing a physician for a considerable time with a variety of somatic complaints. No organic cause evident, he had been placed on every known antianxiety drug without success.

He respected and admired his father, who he felt had always been quite reasonable with him. He described his mother as one who tended to press him to action, to which he would respond with stubborn resistance, and she, in turn, with the silent treatment. He felt that his parents had not exercised undue pressure on him in regard to a career, and that, if they had, it would not have been very useful anyway. His relationship with his sister was always good. She was married and living in another part of the country.

My impression after the preliminary interview was that this was a slender, sensitive, honest, somewhat soft man. His experience abroad had introduced him to "masculine" activities, which he continued to enjoy but which did not seem to lessen his dependent conflicts. A second preliminary interview was arranged.

In the second interview, further information made it possible for me to pose to him the reasons for his coming to me, my understanding of his total situation, and then my offer of a treatment agreement. I told him that he had conveyed to me his concern about the following:

— Time—that his age and place in life were crowding him to make decisions for assuming responsibility for the conduct of his own life
— That he was conflicted, ambivalent about his wish and fear to grow up
— That this, then, included a fear of failure as well as a fear of success
— That he then establishes reasons in advance for not trying and that these reasons are his fear of flying and his fear of people
— That he frequently feels too ill to be able to progress effectively, although he knows that he has no diagnosed physical illness
— That if he fails in graduate school, draft into the service awaits him, and he fears failure in the service, that he will get "sick" there
— That he feels as if his parents have never really allowed him to be self-responsible despite their encouraging him to go abroad for a year after high school

I proposed that we meet twelve times, one hour each time, and that we would direct our attention to two issues so closely related as to be one in fact—that the time would be spent around the problem of his fear of growing up and his fear of success. He was told the exact date of the last interview, and a fee was set. He was told that if it turned out that these were not the issues most important to him, we would know it and would move on to whatever else it was that was more important. He was asked for his agreement to the proposal and his response was affirmative. This was an instance where the patient's time in the geographical area was limited, so that the schedule of interviews was first once each week and later twice each week.

First Interview

He felt better, but quickly complained about the effects he had suffered from having had just one ounce of liquor. He had been dizzy, sick to his stomach, and the next day had had a hangover and a general sense of malaise. He wants to be able to drink freely. Dizziness and nausea had first appeared two years earlier when he was about to leave on a cross-country trip with his parents. He recalled being sick all through the trip. He was convinced that he had syphillis and then decided it must be leukemia. On his return home he felt better. Shortly thereafter he left for another state and got a job as a bus boy for about six weeks. He felt fine until about one week before returning home when the nausea and dizziness became so bad that he went to the emergency room of a nearby hospital three consecutive nights. Nothing was found to account for his symptoms, and he was given a phenothiazine and sleeping pills. I raised the question as to how many men his age spent summers traveling with their parents when he told me that he had traveled with them the previous summer, also. He agreed that it was rather unusual. I remarked that such trips are certainly attractive, but that we must look more closely at them. I asked him to go back in his mind and tell me how it was decided that he spend a year abroad after high school. This was done, he said, to help him grow up, settle down, and be ready for college. Meanwhile he could have the advantage of learning a foreign language. He wanted to go to a prep school in this country and did not wish to go abroad. Moreover, he had a girl for the first time and had enjoyed his senior year at high school. However, he raised no objections to his parents plans for him. His parents went abroad with him, saw to it that he was settled at the school there, and left him. He attended classes very briefly, and on the day that he wrote to his parents saying that he was thinking of leaving that town for another, larger one in Europe, he actually packed and left. He did not attend school for the rest of the year, and his parents never actually pressed him as to what he did abroad. At one point, he made reservations to fly home, but he stuck it out and felt that he had matured socially.

I remarked that few boys at age seventeen would have stuck it out the way he did, that he had certainly made gains, but that his behavior since then made me wonder whether the cure might be worse than the disease. He said he hadn't thought of it that way, and that he had not been conscious of objections to being so closely tied to his parents. He agreed that we might look further into this. I noted for myself that he appeared at ease in the interview and seemed free with me, but displayed a degree of not caring, of apathy, that suggested more depression than he knew of.

Second Interview

The patient did not appear. When it was certain that he was not coming, I called and succeeded in reaching him by phone. He had mistakenly noted our appointment as being the next day. He had actually written the wrong date into his appointment book. He said that he would come to the next regularly scheduled interview, which would be three days later.

He came on time and immediately opened with the news that he had been accepted for a summer course in a specialized subject at a university which was rated best in the subject. However, if he is accepted for the same course at another university near to where his sister lives, he will go to that one. His parents have already decided to drive him out to whichever university he chooses.

He had felt awful the day before. Perhaps it was due to his being with his girl instead of studying. Or, more likely, because he is physically ill in some way. I asked if his mother was a worrier. He said she was, and that he is just like her. Then he spoke of his sense of weakness, including a total physical inadequacy. I pointed out that his interest in sports tells us that there is another side to this feeling about himself. This stimulated him to tell of his always being uncoordinated, even through high school. Nevertheless, he persisted in playing basketball and tackle football with his friends and enjoyed the contact in football. It made him feel tough, like a man. Quickly then he reverted to his fears. Enroute to the interviews he rode the elevated and was afraid that it would jump the tracks and topple to the street. He always sits in the elevated car frightened that he will panic before anything even happens. In order to control this, he sits near an exit so that he will be able to escape. He recognized his even greater fear of being helpless.

I told him that there was a side of him that wanted very much to be different from how he consciously feels about himself (thinking of his fantasies in which he sees himself scoring touchdowns as he watches football on TV, for example), but that something happens to frighten him off—so much so that it is less dangerous to do nothing. Not studying can be less dangerous for him than studying. I related his attachment to his family as a way that he feels controlled, to which he promptly responded with a comment about his "trepidation" about going to summer school alone, in opposition to the wish of his parents. He would need a darned good excuse to get away with that. I said that being in his twenties was sufficient excuse, and he understood. He indicated that his fears and complaints and attachment to his family have always been with him, but had become much worse since his return from abroad. He made it a point to write down the date of our next appointment before leaving the interview. On his way out, he engaged me in a brief conversation about professional basketball and asked if I was interested in it.

Third Interview

He had been thinking about our discussions, and he is not so sure that he is that much attached to his parents. Shortly thereafter, he undid this objection by reminding himself that on nights when he doesn't have a car for his use, one of his parents will pick him up at the public transport station in order to spare him the one mile walk to the house. He "chickened out" today when asked by an instructor to substitute in a class for him. Nothing really matters, since he will be drafted anyway, and there he will chicken out by becoming sick. I said that all of his complaints were saying the same thing, namely, that he was afraid, and that we should see what might be responsible for that. He regards himself as immature and doesn't like to accept responsibility. We moved to the subject of self-esteem, during which discussion I took the position that a man of his age would undoubtedly feel much better about himself if he did something to contribute to his own support, like by getting a job. He responded by agreeing that he *probably* should work and be independent to some degree. He does feel that he is stubborn, but he is also the kind, he says, who yields to others.

It was my own impression that his enormous passivity and his acceptance of it served both to control his destiny and to help him avoid competition and the dangers of success.

Fourth Interview

He had felt somewhat better after the last interview. He reviewed his experience at a college fraternity where he wanted responsibility in running the affairs of the fraternity, but behaved so irresponsibly that he was actually asked to leave. We spoke of his conflict between accepting responsibility for himself and the fear of it, with the end result one of immobility. I remarked on his apathetic presentation of himself. He said that he is bored and depressed, although he knows that there is also present a good deal of optimism and curiosity. After this confession of the more aggressive side of himself, I again took initiative in respect to discussing his need for greater self-esteem and ways of getting it. He became restless and suddenly pulled out his sunglasses and put them on. I raised the question of his placing a barrier between us as a way of keeping me off. He said that he chain-smoked cigarettes without inhaling for the same reason. On his way out I handed him a bill.

Fifth Interview

He was feeling quite good. Earlier in the day, he had raised his hand to speak in class just as soon as it was announced that the subject for discussion was "the academic revolution." The instructor had called on someone else, and he was glad because he had already begun to feel his heart racing, throat constricting, and his body almost incoordinate. All these manifestations of fear were brought to his attention as fear. He is afraid to make independent moves because they have the meaning of "head on" clashes. He would so much prefer something like hypnosis or a pill to quiet his inner turmoil. I elaborated on this as further evidence of his fear to make moves, fear to assume responsibility, and his preference to let someone take over, do it for him and to him. He responded to this by saying that he really trusts machines more than he does people. In riding the elevated, the greatest danger is that the motorman will go too fast, not that there is anything wrong with the cars. In the same way, pilot error is far more dangerous in planes than are any machine errors. Before the interview was ended, we had established that he is afraid, that it has to do with emotional reactions rather than intellectual awareness. On the way out he reminds me that he is really feeling much better. I remind myself that we come to the midpoint in the next interview.

Sixth Interview

He expects trouble at home over the coming weekend because a group of old college friends are coming to his home along with some girls. They will have a big party with lots of alcohol, and his mother will be upset. He is terribly concerned over the fact that he wants to be able to drink a lot without getting such bad hangovers as he had been getting from such very small amounts of alcohol. Drinking is a manifestation of manliness; if he can't drink much it clearly reflects on his masculinity. Last week, for the first time in many months, he went to a restaurant with his girl. He got through it but felt awful. His fear was that he would be seen by others in the restaurant as having shaking hands, being uncoordinated. He feels self-conscious about standing alone in any public place. He wonders if he is effeminate. No, he has no homosexual desires, but he does "torture" himself with thoughts about it. I formulated the situation as one that as a senior in high school he finally got to kiss a girl; then in the year abroad, he learned how to have a woman sexually; these, along with gonorrhea and drinking, made him feel more manly. However, although these served his need at that time, they no longer suffice; now he has to do something more in order to assure himself of his own adequacy.

Seventh Interview

The weekend had gone badly. Prior to the arrival of the many guests for the party, he had been sick to his stomach but had not vomited. When the weekend party broke up, he had felt terribly nostalgic. He would not see any of his special gang of four friends again. They were off to jobs, Vietnam, and other places. He was aware that job, marriage, and responsibility were all before him, and here he is so preoccupied with his adequacy in all these areas. Did I think that he was effeminate? Is he sterile? He recalled the episode of gonorrhea and his later worry about syphillis. Syphillis causes insanity. I talked to him about the effect of gonorrhea on a young boy who gets this infection after his first try at sex and how often it carries the meaning of punishment for his sinful efforts at being a man, particularly in view of the values and codes of conduct of his own background. I added that nevertheless, fear of gonorrhea and of syphillis had not stopped him from seeking and having further sexual experiences, that this was pretty good evidence that his desire to be a man was certainly there, but that he was afraid of it.

I noted to myself that for the first time he had come dressed rather trimly, with a shirt, tie, and coat.

Eighth Interview

He started right out with the statement that he knows now what his problem is, that "we really have hit it," so what does he do now.

"How many meetings do we have left?"

"I don't know."

"Guess."

"Two—this is the eighth."

"How many do we have altogether?"

"Ten."

"I can see why you raised the question that you did even more now. You misunderstood. We have twelve meetings, but you already feel that we are just about at the end and what will you do then."

We discussed his future plans, which remain vague for him. He has no special interest. He does feel better and has not been taking any tranquilizers. He feels that he has to confront the situations he fears and master them. I agree with him and share his confidence that he can do that. He then tells of having gone out to dinner with a group, how he had felt nervous and sick to his stomach for about fifteen minutes and then was over it. Again he returned to his fear of exploiting his potential ability because he feels moved to remain attached and dependent, that dependency holds him down.

Ninth Interview

The end looms nearer and the chips are down. He has been sick to his stomach, he has a cold, the flu, his joints ache—maybe he has arthritis and will be crippled and unable to move. He is depressed, morose, bored. He is too afraid to die, so suicide is out. All these symptoms have flared up since our last meeting. I moved, then, into the area of his being disappointed, reminding him that his expectations of what he would get out of this are rapidly disappearing. I asked him to consider the fact that he might be angry with me and that he is protecting himself from his feelings by developing symptoms. He said that he does become angry on certain issues: (1) The Arabs have been mistreated in the Israeli-Arab situation; the Christ-

ians have made amends to the Jews by taking it out on the Arabs.
(2) In general, he is for the Vietnam war on moral grounds of commitment. (3) He is "violently" against capital punishment. In these issues we see his inner life reflected. In the first, his father is an active, practicing Christian and his therapist is Jewish. The patient is a passively resisting non-Christian. In the second issue, his father is "violently" against the Vietnam war. In the third issue, his father has reservations about such punishment. The patient's enormous concern about capital punishment centers about it as a situation of utter helplessness and his fear of that. He described himself as a "leech." I remarked that such a description must depress him. I reviewed with him the fact that he is now in a battle with me and will probably feel even worse.

Tenth Interview

The preceding week had gone well until about noon on this day when he began to experience some dizziness and nausea. We were able to relate this to his coming to see me today, and his fear of my disapproval. I suggested that this was directly linked with his fear of authority figures. He recalled his fear of going to a prekindergarten play school and that he had forced his withdrawal. He remembered being afraid to go to elementary school and his fear of being apart from his mother and home. I related all these to his coming today. I said that this was a rather vivid demonstration of his concern that if he is well, I will send him away, and that if he is sent away, it must carry the meaning for him that he is not loved and certainly found to be unacceptable. He tells of his "trepidation" about telling his parents that he has decided to take an incomplete in one course until he turns in a paper. We discuss how he will go about telling his professor of his decision. He fears the professor's censure. He then revealed that his first inclination was to tell the professor that he was ill, emotionally upset and in psychiatric treatment.

Eleventh Interview

He had had a six-pack of beer the night before and had a headache this morning which is still present slightly. Beer and alcohol are ways of lessening his sensitivity to rebuff. I remind him that if alcohol can do this for him, then he has the capacity to manage this without it. The matter of rebuff opened the question of his feelings and fear of being unacceptable as an old fear of not being wanted by his parents, and how he now has this feeling with me, particularly so since we are coming to the end of treatment. He tells me of some of his daydreams—he is building a city; he sees a car that he likes and is driving it; he is in the "field" with a gun. I remarked on the activity in all these fantasies and how much they told us what he wanted but feared lest he be turned away. I added that he has employed a general pattern of being unobtrusive so as not to draw attention to himself by his behavior or by his dress, that he wants to lay low and then maybe he will be wanted. He agreed with this, and I reviewed the coming end of treatment with him, that he will regard it as a rejection, that I don't care for him and don't want him. He replied that he did believe that I had given him only twelve sessions because I did not think he was deserving of more. I asked him if it had occurred to him that I had offered him only twelve because I knew that he had the stuff to do something for himself? He had not. I repeated my confidence in him.

Twelfth Interview

He had told his father that he was taking an incomplete in one course until he turned in a paper. Father was angry and had told mother, who was also angry. He had to cancel an invitation to a cookout and was very nervous out of his fear that his friend would condemn and reject him. He feels that his major concern is the fear of rejection, that he is worthless. I went into this with him actively in respect to termination and separation. He had thought much about this last meeting and found himself thinking that he would ask me for a number of guidelines. Then he realized that I would not give them to him and that he could do it for himself. He is aware that he has allowed events to impose decisions on him rather than taken action to shape events. He has found himself thinking about the uselessness of everything, of being depressed, and his need to carry on on his own and be independent. He raised a number of questions, such as what will he do if he remains anxious in a restaurant, or feels sick. I went into this as being only a plea for more from me. He then realized how different things are for him now as compared to when he started with me. He has some feelings of disappointment, but he will be able to manage those. I told him that he should not take the end of treatment as a rejection, meaning that he is unworthy, nor should he be surprised if he has unkind thoughts about me, and I assured him that if he has such thoughts they should be acceptable to him, since they are to me. He told of his plans for the immediate future, and I reminded him that to do for himself was most important, and that the approval of parents, of me, or of anyone else should be secondary to his own wish to do for himself. As he is about to leave, he tells me that his parents are buying a car for him so that he can drive out to his summer course himself. He doesn't fully like the idea of their getting a car for him, and I suggested that he can always pay them off for it if he so wishes.

Follow-up Six Months after Termination

He looks very good with a trim beard and moustache that he grew during the summer session he had attended at the university distant from his sister. He had had no problems with eating with others and had worked hard. He had become depressed in the last week of his stay there, and it had continued for a week after returning home. He is aware that this is a familiar pattern. On one occasion during that summer, he had felt sick, went to a physician who found nothing, so he "forgot" about it and has been well since. He is now engaged to the girl he had been seeing during his visits with me, and his parents approved of this step. He is planning his graduate work so that he will be able to gain entry to a prestigious school for his doctoral work. He worries about the draft now, but only because he feels guilty about not wishing to serve. He has come to an anti-Vietnam position. He expects to marry the next summer and dreads doing that and promptly being drafted. He does a lot of beer drinking and continues to worry about its effects on his liver. Although uncertain about his future career, he is confident that he can teach. He would like to earn a lot of money, and that reminds him that he is still afraid to fly and that he may one day need help with that. It is apparent that his social anxiety is greatly diminished and that there is considerable increase in his self-esteem. He looks more mature and more confident. Somatic problems are minimal. He was pleased to see me, is able to use the insights he gained, and, most of all, seemed clearly to understand that he can be independent even if by steps at a time.

Follow-up One Year after Termination

He looks neat, well-dressed, and handsome with his goatee and moustache. He is getting married next week. He has gotten his Master's degree and is awaiting admission to other schools for work on his doctorate in a specialized field. He is very much aware of his dependent desires and his inclination to yield to them. He feels that his social anxiety is enormously diminished and that in some ways he is definitely more aggressive. Most of all he recognizes his problems and is aware that it is only he who can master them. When he worries about illness and the effects on his liver, he knows that he wants to have all his needs gratified and to give up none. He feels that he is making slow progress, but progress, toward accepting the limitations on gratification that reality and independence demand. He looks it, too. He remains very much aware of the major issues that we talked about.

Postscript

Almost exactly one year later, two years after the end of treatment, a chance encounter with his mother brought from her the unsolicited information that a "miracle" had been worked on her son and that he was doing very well in work, marriage, and independence.

6 The Selection of Patients

Choosing the most appropriate kind of treatment for a particular psychiatric patient is often a most vexing and difficult problem. It is less difficult only in those cases in which illness is so overtly severe as to make clear the need for immediate intervention and where the means for intervention are limited in number. For example, profound depression will require active drug therapy, or, depending on the age of the patient, electric shock treatment, or both. Similarly, the acutely disturbed schizophrenic patient or the manic patient will immediately suggest the use of chemical means for alleviating the condition. It is in the vast majority of nonpsychotic patients or in the not inconsiderable numbers of nonacutely disturbed psychotic patients where the proper choice of treatment presents many puzzles. One simple solution is to adopt the method of the behavior therapists (or the behavior modification therapists), who choose as their target in all cases the single presenting symptom that troubles the patient. Thus, it is the patient's anxiety attacks, or his phobia, or his sexual deviation that is attacked without regard for any one or more of the unconsciously derived determinants that have entered into the formation of the symptom or of the behavior.

There are a very few guidelines for the accurate choice of treatment (and therefore for the accurate selection of patients for particular treatment) in all instances in which treatment is individualized in accord with the best judgment as to the patient's needs. In practice, this means that it is in the selection of patients for exploratory psychotherapy, whether long or short, that refined criteria for treatment are most urgently needed. It means further that the greatest difficulties in treatment choice arise when one prefers to employ a treatment method that aims at making possible for the patient to arrive for himself at a position where previously unknown options will be available to him.

Accurate nosological diagnosis in psychiatry in no way illuminates the unique life history of the individual. Nor does it convey any sense of the adaptive ego strengths of the patient, of his achievements, and, most significantly, of the precise nature of his capacity to effect object relationships.

The selection of patients for any short form of psychotherapy includes an additional hazard not present if long-term therapy is prescribed. It is common experience, as much for the experienced psychotherapist or psychoanalyst as for the inexperienced, that an initial diagnosis and treatment prescription is found to be grossly inappropriate once treatment is in progress over some relatively short period of time. The extent to which a patient is a borderline psychotic, or frankly psychotic, or overtly homosexual, or alcoholic, or drug addicted, for example, may sometimes be discovered only after treatment has begun. The skill that some people have for concealment occurs sufficiently often so as to keep the most astute of clinicians and diagnosticians humble. In long-term psychotherapy, there is the opportunity over time to come to an accurate diagnosis which validates the kind of treatment already begun, signals a change in the method or goals of treatment, or indicates a completely different therapeutic regime. In any of the short forms of psychotherapy, the brevity of the treatment obviously demands even sharper delineation of its suitability for this kind of patient. Even more is this the case in psychotherapy in which time itself is specifically limited. It has already been noted that one of the steps in arranging the treatment agreement with the patient is to mention that if it soon turns out that the chosen central issue is, in fact, not at all central, then patient and therapist will know it and will make a change to the more salient issue. In practice, the strict limitation of time demands even closer attention to the selection of the correct central issue, since any change in the focus of attention after the first one or two treatment meetings already seriously reduces the amount of time available to the patient for his treatment.

It may be readily noted that the selection of a central issue or focus is very different from making an accurate dynamic diagnosis. The chronic alcoholic patient may present himself for treatment on the basis of very troublesome marital relations and conceal totally the fact of his alcoholism. The therapist may choose the marital relationship as the central issue only to discover the alcoholism midway or beyond in treatment. Or, a homosexual patient may project as the central issue his embattled relationships with employers or other authority figures. Neither of these situations, or others like it, needs to be taken as a contraindication to the continuation of treatment, since treatment may continue not with the relief of the alcoholism as the issue but rather with the marital problem as the continuing focus of treatment, or not with the homosexuality as the issue but rather the difficulties with authority figures. From the nature of the therapeutic process described here, it may not be too much to expect that adherence to the central issue, even when confronted by the discovery of a widespread personality disorder, will lead to greater self-awareness in respect to the personality disorder and will influence, to some degree, positive change in the patient, even in respect to the larger personality problem.

The critic may now state, in all fairness, that I have moved from a position that called for razor-sharp diagnosis because of the severe time limitation to a position that says that any person can be treated by the method simply by choosing a reasonably correct central issue and clinging to it. In this instance, both the critic and the author are correct. The sharper the diagnosis of the patient's disorder, the more accurate the selection by the therapist of the central issue. However, since the statement of the central issue is often global and becomes increasingly sharpened in the course of the twelve meetings, it means that even the less accurate diagnostic assessment still allows for patient and therapist to begin with a somewhat less sharply defined, global central issue. In other words, accurate diagnosis as a means of selecting patients for this mode of treatment is less important, with some few exceptions, than the selection of a central issue and the skill in conducting the treatment. The exceptions have already been noted: the patient so severely depressed as to be unable to negotiate, let alone tolerate, a treatment agreement; the patient in an acute psychotic state; and the patient whose desperation in life centers exclusively around the need for and the incapacity to tolerate object relations. The last exception requires further definition, since the term *borderline* is too much a diagnostic wastebasket.

With critical emphasis placed on the degree to which separation-individuation has been mastered and the test of both the extent of mastery and the capacity for further growth entering decisively in the termination phase of treatment, it is likely that the most serious possibility for inflicting psychological damage in this treatment method could occur from the failure to recognize a patient as belonging to the so-called borderline group and, further, what kind of border-line the patient is. The work of Kernberg and of Grinker and his colleagues have served to clarify the varieties of conditions that may be subsumed under the heading borderline syndrome.[1] Within the syndrome, there is a range of patients who share the same dynamic ego defects but whose ultimate personality organization varies in

1. O. Kernberg, "Borderline Personality Organization," *Journal of the American Psychoanalytic Association*, 15 (1967), 641; R. R. Grinker, B. Werble, and R. C. Drye, *the Borderline Syndrome* (New York: Basic Books, 1968).

accordance with variations in the intensity of the ego defects. Grinker distinguishes four general varieties within the borderline syndrome, ranging from the psychotic border, in patients with the most serious incapacity to promote object relationships, to the fourth group, the border with the neurosis, in patients with obvious greater capacity to the extent that they may more often be recognized as severe neurotic character disorders. He describes four basic ego dysfunctions as characteristic of the borderline syndrome: (1) Anger as the main or only affect experienced; (2) defective affectional relationships which are anaclitic, dependent, or complementary, but rarely reciprocal; (3) no indications of consistent self-identity; and (4) depression—more as loneliness and lack of commitment than of despair. Skillful diagnosis in the intake or consultative interviews, understanding always that these may be extended until one arrives at some certainty in respect to the diagnosis, makes it possible to select from among the borderline syndrome group patients who will be suitable for treatment. In the absence of certainty, it is probably better to exclude such patients.

Sifneos uses a set of specific criteria for determining the suitability for treatment.[2] These include evidence of superior academic functioning or work performance; at least one meaningful relationship with another person during his lifetime; ability to interact with the evaluating psychiatrist by expressing some affect during the interview; a specific complaint . Also, some determination is made of the patient's motivation for psychotherapy. These criteria are, to a certain extent, a rough guide for the recognition and exclusion of the borderline patients.

Restriction to those with superior academic or work performance does not apply in this method of time-limited psychotherapy. Actually, there is some evidence to show that the specificity of the treatment, with its concrete, prescriptionlike qualities, brings it closely within the experience of patients from lower socio-economic groups, so that they can engage in it successfully so long as some average or reasonable degree of intelligence is present. The limited duration of treatment and the intensity of involvement generated by the treatment process serve also to counteract the often noted reluctance of many of the lower socio-economic group to engage in talk treatment. The separation-individuation process and the problems arising from it spare no human being; middle- or upper-class experiences are not necessary to make a patient suitable for this kind of psychotherapy.

Sifneos' requirement that the patient must have a specific complaint can be qualified in this method. The selection of a focus or

2. P. E. Sifneos, "Short-Term, Anxiety-provoking Psychotherapy: An Emotional Problem-Solving Technique," *Seminars in Psychiatry*, I, no. 4 (November 1969).

central issue may be more readily obtained in instances in which the patient does have a specific complaint around which the evaluating interview may be used to determine whether it will be the central issue, or whether the specific complaint is the derived expression of a more cogent but concealed central issue. Some patients are unable to present themselves with a specific complaint, suffering as they do with a mixture of feelings and thoughts that emerge in consciousness as a vague sense of unease, shadowy anxiety, or uncertain discontent. In the course of the preliminary interviews, it is usually possible to gain the kind of information which allows then for patient and therapist to arrive at a specific complaint. If a patient does not present with a specific complaint, and if in the preliminary interviews it is still not possible to arrive at one, this in itself may be taken as a contraindication to treatment. In such instances, this may be a clue to the presence of a severe borderline state or a chronic, undifferentiated schizophrenic state in which there is no motivation for change but rather the ambiguous longing for total passive, narcissistic gratification.

Jacob Swartz, Director of the Psychiatry Clinic at University Hospital of Boston University Medical Center, in reviewing his experience in adopting the twelve-hour treatment plan, believes that the criteria for selection of patients are not remarkably different from the selection of patients for any kind of psychotherapy that will be offered in an out-patient clinic. He feels that the ability to delineate a focus of treatment is more important than diagnostic category as a criterion for selection of patients.[3]

There is a very large group of patients for whom the twelve hour treatment plan is admirably suited, even indicated. Young men and women, roughly in middle or late adolescence, mostly college students, who present themselves with any of a multitude of psychological and somatic complaints make up the majority of this group. In the absence of the few severe disqualifying conditions, it is likely that the patient is in the midst of a maturational crisis. There is no question but that this general category of disorder is the most common in this age group. The particular pressures and strains of college life, with its attendant problems related to career, independence, identity, and so forth confront each student with almost daily challenges to his growth and development as a responsible, interacting, relating adult. The emotional upsets that appear are exquisitely related to the separation-individuation process, and the degree of flexibility usually present in these young people makes the termination phase of the treatment a genuine growth-consolidating experience. The patient in a maturational crisis is best served by treatment that engages all of his own inclinations toward maturity. Hence, a

3. J. Swartz, "Time-Limited Brief Psychotherapy," *Seminars in Psychiatry*, I, no. 4 (November 1969).

time limit addresses itself to his desire for independence and the confidence that the time is sufficient for him to do the job that must be done. The choice of a central issue is for him the unambiguous task and goal. To these are added all the unconscious wishes and fantasies that will be slowly sacrificed to the demands of reality and adulthood within the active relationship promoted by the therapist between patient and therapist.

Any kind of definitive answers as to the selection of patients for any kind of therapy, psychotherapy, behavior therapy, or drug therapy can only come from the combination of a vast amount of accumulated clinical experience and observation along with the application of increasingly rigorous research methods that will dissect and tease out the significant factors and variables involved. Scientific studies that center around the reactions of people, one to another, must be rigorous, but can never be interpreted in their results as we would pure laboratory studies. The varieties of interaction that are possible defy imagination, and it is not due to lack of effort that outcome studies of all kinds of psychiatric treatment are notoriously uncertain.

One of the potentially rich byproducts of this method of time-limited psychotherapy is that by strictly defining its duration and by elaborating clear-cut guidelines for the conduct of the treatment based upon clear-cut exposition of the concurrent dynamic process, it may be possible for both clinicians and researchers in many places to come closer to studying the same thing than in any other kind of psychotherapy. McNair remarks as follows: "A fixed time limit has another advantage beyond the greater simplicity of brevity . . . Usually, there is great variation in both the number of interviews and the duration of treatment. The ending point is some joint function of the therapist's and patient's interpretation of the results . . . Fixing the time limits not only brings the treatment within a practical period for research, but it also is a major step toward quantifying and bringing under experimental control the amount of treatment administered. In drug study jargon, time limits are analagous to fixed dosage schedules. With better quantitative measurements of additional aspects of the treatment and more research, we may even be able to sketch some answers to fixed dosage of what?"[4]

McNair addresses himself to only two factors that will enormously facilitate research into selection, process, and outcome—the brevity and the exact time limit. The treatment method itself, with its treatment agreement, the sequence of dynamic events, and the participation of the therapist offer additional standards and rationale for all other clinicians and researchers to attempt, follow, observe, record, modify, and refine.

4. D. M. McNair, "A Season for Brevity," *Seminars in Psychiatry*, I, no. 4 (November 1969).

7 Teaching This Treatment Method

The introduction of any new treatment method is commonly met with skepticism, questions and, at best, with reserved enthusiasm. These are not unexpected, and as the method is brought into use, observations and information as to its assets and liabilities are shared, so that in time some degree of concensus is established as to the effectiveness of the treatment method. The very nature of psychiatry, directed as it is to the emotional problems of each patient and being a field in which, in contrast to other branches of medicine, the physician cannot conceal his own anxieties in a mass of laboratory data and technical procedures, readily stimulates controversy and polarization about any new method. Discussion about the method is often cogent and useful; controversy generally connotes the presence of heat, of emotional positions that stand behind and motivate the presumably logical contentions that are being made. Resistance to a treatment method, to any treatment method, is to be expected on the grounds of rational inquiry. In psychiatry, with very few exceptions of which none come to mind, there is always resistance to any new treatment concept, and in every case, the resistance clearly includes the same meaning as the phenomenon of mental functioning observed so readily in the treatment of all patients. Thus, much and even all of the objection to a particular therapeutic mode may derive from the personal need to avoid the undoing of a fantasy both precious and important to the psychic economy of the antagonist. The other extreme is the psychiatrist who plunges with exuberance and enthusiasm into any new scheme in the hope that it will make possible the fulfillment of a preciously held fantasy. As a result, it is usually insufficient to introduce a new treatment method, particularly if it incorporates some unusual innovations, by proposing that it be tried in a modest way and given the test of application and outcome. The emotional resistances to it are apt to foreclose a fair trial, since it will seem in the best personal interests of those so involved to make certain that it will fail.

The time-limited treatment method developed here will also meet with resistance of this nature, so that any discussion about teaching the method must begin with some exploration of some of the resistances that are aroused in response to this particular variety of psychotherapy.

The experienced therapist is apt to be pessimistic as to what can be achieved in the time available. His involvement with patients in longer forms of psychotherapy has demonstrated the enormous complexities and subtleties of human conflict. Moreover, he has had ample evidence for the multi-determination of symptomatic and character-ologic neurotic disorders. On theoretical grounds, he will find much with which to disagree. Separation-individuation as the final common pathway will seem to him to be too simplistic on the one hand, and too much placing all problems into a common mold. He will find the selection of a central issue interesting, but too restrictive to expect that concentration on the one issue can lead to any kind of satisfying resolution. He will not believe that it will be possible for an intense transference situation to develop so rapidly, nor will he believe that the dynamic events can appear so clearly and so swiftly. It will follow logically in his thinking that this being so, it would hardly be likely that the termination period could induce a powerful reaction in the patient and be a powerful instrument for resolution for both patient and therapist. Finally, having become long used to his own method of treatment, he will be naturally resistive to exposing himself to the learning of a new, seemingly unconventional treatment modality. Failing all these arguments, the experienced therapist will turn his concern to the patient and decry the method as one that short-changes the patient; by this he will mean that the patient is not being given enough, since what we know about the genesis and process of emotional disorders demands that every patient be given "the full treatment."

The inexperienced therapist may manifest his resistance paradoxically. He may adopt the method with enthusiasm and unbounded zeal in his search and need for quick cures. This is particularly likely in the period of transition from medical school and internship, with their emphasis on physical methods of diagnosis and treatment, to the atmosphere of the psychiatric ward or clinic, where there are far greater ambiguities in respect to both diagnosis and treatment. The challenge of psychiatry in general and of psychotherapy in particular to the new therapist is not only that he will have to tolerate even more ambiguity than he had experienced in other branches of medicine, but that he must give up the hope of effecting rapid and specific cures, limited as even these may be in medicine in general. The introduction of a specific type of psychotherapy may arouse his hopes that psychiatry can be like other medical specialties. At the heart of this expectation is the renewed expectation that omnipotence will once more be his. With this set of mind, the inexperienced therapist will place too much reliance on the structure of the treatment process and will quickly run afoul of the patient's disappointment as the doctor's magic and the patient's magical expectations begin to fail. The greater the reliance of the therapist on irrational expectations of the treatment method, the more subject is he to disappointment in himself, which is quickly turned on to the treatment method in an understandable defensive move. Of equal importance in considering the role and participation of the inexperienced therapist is that the lure of quick cure may serve him as a means of avoiding the complicated, anxious, and difficult exchange that arises between patient and therapist in long-term psychotherapy or in psychoanalysis. He may avoid thereby what is to be learned about human behavior in depth and over time, so that he will miss out on the essential ingredients that enter into the making of a psychiatrist—or the making of anyone whose aim it is to be an expert in individual human behavior.

Both experienced and inexperienced therapists may oppose the method by posing still other objections which are in the nature of rationalizations designed to avoid the major emotional objections— that is, anxiety about entering into an intense relationship not only of short duration but of a fixed duration, and anxiety that much of the success of the treatment will depend upon the therapist remaining firm with the conditions of the treatment agreement with the necessity for dealing actively with the separation process. One of the ways in which all therapists may sustain both their own dependent needs as well as their need to have others dependent upon them is to prolong treatment within the framework of the institutionalized setting and thereby prolong the patient's need for the therapist. This is but another expression of the unconscious need for all physicians, for all the so-called helping professions, to exercise socially and morally acceptable control over others. The therapist's own anxieties over separation tend to be experienced in indentification with the patient. As a result, even though in actual practice the therapist is exercising considerable control over the patient in limiting exactly the duration of treatment, such control dims entirely in the face of anxiety over termination that is known from the start. It is this issue that will most contribute to expressions of lack of confidence about being able to do the required task in so short a time or that the method can possibly work.

With awareness of the various resistances that are certain to arise, we may move on to the manner of teaching its conduct. An ideal method is for a therapist who is experienced with this treatment scheme to treat a patient while being observed through a one-way mirror, or on closed-circuit television. Discussions should be held with the therapist and all observers both before and after the treatment sessions. The observers may serve as students of the therapist as well as supervisors of his work from the advantage of their uninvolved position. This kind of teaching plan is useful, too, where none of the therapists has had any experience with the method. The requirement would be that the therapist who will treat a patient while being observed be skilled, experienced, and well versed in psychoanalytically oriented psychotherapy. The only other requirement might be courage, since many therapists are sensitively averse to having others watch them at work.

The key to successful teaching and learning in any kind of psychotherapy lies in the supervisory process. The therapist gaining experience in this method must be carefully supervised at each step of the way. This means that he should consult with his supervisor in respect to each of the twelve treatment meetings as well as in connection with the preliminary interview(s) and in the establishment of the treatment agreement. The supervisor must pay close attention to each detail of the treatment agreement and take nothing for granted. One will find all too often that the therapist has somehow forgotten to inform the patient of the termination date; or has let it be known to the patient that the termination date need not be taken too seriously. In other instances, the therapist may fail to communicate clearly a central issue; or he may fail to elicit the patient's agreement or disagreement with the treatment plan. At the risk of being labelled rigid and compulsive, the supervisor must bring into discussion each detail of the treatment agreement. Failure to do so will serve to minimize the importance of the details for the therapist, and, if the details have been omitted or distorted with the patient, the treatment sessions to follow will very likely fail of their goal.

Supervisory discussions prior to the meeting in which the therapist arranges the treatment agreement are especially useful as a means of teaching and learning the selection of a central issue from the historical data already obtained from the patient. Obviously, a good deal of experience is necessary for one to be able to sort out the data obtained and extract one issue, global or specific, which is central in the present circumstance of the patient and runs through his previous life history.

Once treatment meetings have begun, the supervisor should follow the therapist in his work of each meeting, keeping in mind the series and sequence of dynamic events described and observing carefully the therapist's ability to spot these events and the manner of his response to them. The supervisor will quickly find that the therapist is likely to forget or avoid the central issue, or to leave the central issue and begin to wander afield. It will be important to help the therapist appreciate the ways in which the central issue can be elaborated in material which is derived from it and not necessarily always directly expressed in the specific terms of the central issue. The therapist's reactions to early improvement followed shortly thereafter by signs of complaint or relapse must be related to the phase of treatment. It will come as no surprise to the supervisor when he finds that the therapist misses gross clues from the patient in relation to the impending end of treatment, or simply ignores the fact of a coming end, or has already signaled a message to the patient that the end is uncertain. Without exception, each therapist beginning in this method has difficulty facing up to the separation-termination as an active, predetermined procedure and needs the most help in mastering that phase of treatment. It is not indicated that the supervisor deal with the therapist's personal anxieties and conflicts about separation; it is usually sufficient that the evidence for the problem be obtained from his dealings with his patient as he is gently but firmly pressed to continue to satisfy the details of the treatment agreement. The defensive rationalizations already noted should be explained for what they are by the supervisor.

From the point of view of process, one will find that close attention to the details of the treatment agreement, the sequence of dynamic events, and the participation of the therapist as described here will serve with rather remarkable clarity to answer questions as to what the patient's dynamic situation is and in which phase he is presently involved. Conducted by a skilled therapist, well in control of his own problems, it is almost impossible not to know exactly where one is with the patient at any given time.

It is evident that this kind of psychotherapy requires a high degree of skill, knowledge, and experience. Knowledge of the psychoanalytic theories of mental functioning heavily buttressed by experience in the long-term treatment of patients is the best preparation for this treatment plan. Short treatment in no way suggests easy treatment. In many ways, short treatment is more difficult than longer treatment, even for the experienced therapist. In this time-limited psychotherapy, the therapist must be able to detect very quickly the messages being signaled by the patient in his verbal communication directly. At the same time, the verbal messages and nonverbal behavior may be even more revealing in their unconscious content, and to these, too, the therapist must be attuned. He must be able to translate very adeptly the unconscious messages into derived, acceptable-to-the-patient questions, comments, or formulations that are at the same time directly related to the central issue. In other words, the skills gained slowly and painfully only by the long, arduous dedication to long-term, psychoanalytically oriented psychotherapy or psychoanalysis provide the essentials for the proper and skillful conduct of this kind of time-limited psychotherapy.

If these are the requirements, how then can one justify teaching this method to psychiatry residents as early as the beginning of their second year of residency? Or teaching the method to other professionals who are exposed to considerably less of the required experience than one finds in the well organized psychiatric residency? With the kind of very close supervision that is suggested from the first preliminary interview through to the last words of the final treatment meeting, and by having the resident read and reread the guidelines, in all their aspects, it is possible to guide the inexperienced resident through this treatment scheme very successfully. Holding fast to the central issue enables the resident to isolate something like a single channel to and from the patient's unconscious. For the same reason, he is able to detect and appreciate more readily the connection and relation between unconscious impulse or fantasy and conscious adaptive, ego operation, so that he is better able to communicate with the patient on the latter level, rather than in unconscious concepts, with their libidinal and aggressive contents. The single focus in the midst of a series of rapidly developing transference events provides a uniquely transparent exposition of the basic phenomena of the unconscious mind in the psychotherapeutic setting. The resident comes to learn that the unconscious is not an abstraction, nor is transference a hazy mystery, nor can termination be lightly dismissed. These are important lessons that will stimulate the curious, inquiring resident to seek opportunity to engage in long-term psychotherapy and in psychoanalysis in order to study these phenomena more closely and follow their ramifications. The less curious and inquiring may settle on this kind of treatment as sufficient for whatever further he will do in psychiatry. In such instances, he must be discouraged from concluding that he has gained sufficient expertise to warrant the expert role of psychiatrist. It is not fair to let him learn of his inadequacies only when he has completed his formal training and works on his own without benefit of supervision.

There is nothing to stop all mental health professionals, regardless of the level of their skills and experience, from employing this method of time-limited psychotherapy, and many poorly qualified therapists will undoubtedly leap eagerly into it. The more thoughtful and more experienced in the field in general will realize that the limitation in time and in goals requires a high order of knowledge and self-discipline in conjunction with a disciplined treatment rationale. Close and repeated study of the rationale and process described here, along with expert supervision at each step in the course of treatment are absolute essentials for growing competence in the therapist and progressive benefits for patients. It is a means for treating a great number of patients in a substantial and meaningful way, and it also offers high promise as an accurate research tool into the process and effectiveness of psychotherapy.

Part Two   *The Case of the*
             Conquered Woman

The Case of the Conquered Woman

The following case illustrates the essential points of the theory of the limitation of time, the rationale for treatment, the conduct of treatment, the sequential development of the dynamic process, and the outcome of treatment. All twelve interviews are included. At key points of the treatment—the beginning, the middle, and the end, for example—only repetitive details are omitted. Other interviews have been edited only where the patient is presenting irrelevant material and where I, the therapist, await the opportunity to move back toward the central issue. Follow-up interviews five months and one and a half years after the termination of treatment are included.

The patient was seen by a second-year resident in the psychiatric clinic and then presented to the director of the clinic staff in a regular intake disposition conference. The director knew that I was looking for a patient to be treated by me with the resident group observing over closed-circuit television. I had asked only that the patient chosen be one who talks and had indicated nothing about diagnosis, age, social status, or the like. At the disposition conference, the decision was made that this might be a suitable patient for a teaching case. The patient was told that she would be treated by Dr. Mann and was asked for her agreement to allow the treatment to be televised so that the other doctors in the clinic could observe. She had no objection to this procedure. I was not present at the disposition conference; my first contact with the patient was, as it turned out, in our first treatment session.

The following information is taken from the resident's intake interview:

The patient is a thirty-nine-year-old, white, Roman Catholic woman, mother of six, referred from the medical clinic. There is no history of previous psychiatric help.

Chief Complaint: "Always afraid something is going to happen."

Present Illness: Patient dated the onset of her fears to ten years ago when, while watching a movie in which a craniotomy was being done, she experienced the onset of sudden difficulties with breathing and became frightened that she was having a heart attack. For the following ten years she has had nightly episodes of waking from her sleep with hot and cold sweats, the feeling that her head was going to split. At around two or three in the morning, she awakens her husband, who is at first understanding, but then becomes angry and causes the patient to cry, after which she feels better and is able to return to sleep.

About six years ago, she began to limit her churchgoing to confession when she began to suffer claustrophobia there (her father died at about this time). She avoids movies for the same reason, and recently her fears have extended so that she doesn't go outdoors for walks with her children.

Her symptoms have become worse since her last baby was born eight months ago, and at present, she is afraid that she may lose control, pass out, and that during her unconsciousness some harm will befall her children. Earlier in the summer of this year, she developed tension headaches and was worked up at this hospital, but no organic cause for them was found. She has gained a good deal of weight in recent months, which she feels is due to her drinking beer at bedtime in order to help herself to sleep.

The patient's husband is embarking on the last of five years of night courses, three times weekly, toward promotion in his present job. She misses him during those evenings.

The patient is the youngest of five children. She describes a relatively strict and restricted life due to the strictness of her father, who did not allow his children to participate in many school events. Menarche began at age ten and was accompanied by migraine headaches attributed to her menses. She was unhappy about menstruating and had dysmennorrhea from the beginning. She engaged in no formal dating until she was seventeen and her first experience with sexual intercourse came with her marriage. She describes her present sex life by saying she can "take it or leave it."

Following high school graduation, she worked as a clerk in a large company and lived at home until she married at age twenty-three. Mother is seventy-five, lives alone a short bus ride from the patient, whom mother rarely visits. She is described as domineering and difficult, and she never approved of any of her children's spouses. She is dependent and demanding of the patient for help with her own practical difficulties. Father died six years ago at age seventy of a heart attack. The death was sudden and the patient was very depressed over the loss. Although strict, he would always come to the patient's house with a bag of candy for the children, and he was the parent with whom the patient felt closest. The parents fought; the father drank considerably, and the patient was of the opinion that all the children were nervous because of the constant arguments in the house.

The patient's oldest child is a fifteen-year-old girl described as an ideal teenager. Next is a thirteen-year-old son who has trouble with his school work; then a ten-year-old daughter who is regularly ill with headaches and stomach pains, so that the patient feels that this girl is very much like herself. There is another daughter, age six, a boy of four who has temper tantrums, and the youngest, a girl of eight months. The patient has had two spontaneous abortions.

In the disposition conference, it was agreed that she was suffering spreading phobic symptoms on the basis of well-repressed aggressive and libidinal strivings, in good measure a result of the oppressive attitude in her parental home. She was assigned for treatment as a teaching case, and a preliminary focus of treatment was suggested to the convened clinic staff but not to the patient: the focus would be to help her accept her conflicting drives, which might be approached through attempts to help her ease her situation with her children so that her adult life would not be so oppressive as had been her childhood. The diagnosis of anxiety neurosis was made.

As a means of formulating a central issue prior to the patient's next visit, during which, if the formulation seemed to hold its validity, the treatment agreement would be negotiated and treatment begun, the following data was extracted from the preliminary interview.

Ten years ago:
    One month of arthritis.
    Sees craniotomy in the movies.
    Anxiety attacks begin at night, and phobic symptoms appear.
    Third child, a daughter, is born. It is this daughter who, among all the children, is described as also having somatic symptoms.
Six years ago:
    Father dies.
    Claustrophobic symptoms appear.
Eight months ago:
    Sixth child, a girl, is born.
    Since then, growing fear of loss of control, passing out, harming her children.

The anxiety attacks and the phobic symptoms are the most prominent disabling symptoms and prompt the psychoanalytic understanding that these are ego defenses operating against dangerous instinctual drives in such a way as to externalize into an outer danger what is unconsciously felt as an inner danger. On this basis, the focus of treatment as proposed in the intake disposition conference was well placed. However, our strategy is not only to avoid exploration of deeply unconscious and vigorously defended fantasies of both libidinal and aggressive nature but, equally important, to present a central issue to the patient which she can understand, consciously, as pertinent to her life, but which is still clearly related to the repressed conflicts and which is recurrent over time and therefore of both genetic and adaptive significance.

We reinterpret the data we have in relation to the outstanding realistic burden in her present life—a burden added to by the related nature of her symptoms. Might it not be too much for her to manage six young children, and might it not be that the link from the past to the present in respect to her neurotic state lies in her relationships with her children and with her husband?

On this basis, I decided that the best way to formulate a central issue that would encompass past and present, be recurrent over time, make sense to the patient, and be available for investigation, treatment, and resolution would be to tell the patient that the problem most troublesome to her at this time is that *she is suffering from a constant sense of nagging discontent, irritation, and irritability.* Clearly this is a global issue, and one that might be true of very many patients presenting themselves with very different complaints. However, the global issue will become more and more defined in the course of treatment; moreover, in this case the global issue has a direct connection with the unconscious neurotic elements that have a life history extending far into the past and emerging directly in the present. If it is a correct formulation, it will make sense and be immediately felt by the patient as valid both consciously and unconsciously.

First Interview

Dr.:   I would like to ask you this: what is there about the way that you are feeling that you would most want to be helped with? (*An immediate focusing effort.*)

Pt.:   The anxiety that I have.

Dr.:   Can you tell me something more about it?

Pt.:   Well, I will get up in the morning and feel alright. My husband will be there, and my children will be there, and I will help everybody get out. Then when everybody is gone I am left with the two little ones. I will try to start my work, and I will feel this anxiety build up and my head will get hot, and then I will feel kind of shaky, and then I feel that I can't control myself and I don't want to be alone. (*She has already accented the burden of her children.*)

Dr.:   Now, do I understand correctly that this has been going on for a long time? (*A move into the history of the present disabling life circumstance.*) . . .

Pt.:   Ten years . . . I was in a movie when this all started and I remembered just when it was, and my daughter is now ten and she was an infant.

Dr.:   What is her name?

Pt.:   Jessica.

Dr.:   Isn't that your name? Your daughter is Jessica and you are Jessica. (*Recalling that it is this child who seems to be most like her mother neurotically.*)

Pt.:   Yes.

Dr.:   How come the same name?

Pt.:   I just thought that I would name one after me. I had to name one after my husband.

Dr.:   Which one is named after him?

Pt.:   My daughter, Davida. She was supposed to have my husband's name, David.

She is the oldest and I thought that if it were a boy it would be David, but I changed it to Davida.

Dr.: You were saying that it began ten years ago when Jessica was born.

Pt.: After she was born. Well, I would say that she was an infant, let's say maybe about six months old.

Dr.: And you went to a movie and what happened?

Pt.: I got very disturbed watching the movie, and I started to have heavy palpitations, and I got scared, and I just walked out.

Dr.: What were you seeing at the movie that was so—

Pt.: It was a medical picture and they were performing head surgery. Of course, I had been to theaters before and had seen all kinds. Probably at that time—

Dr.: You might have been especially tense or nervous at that time?

Pt.: Probably. Well, I was having trouble with arthritis at the same time. I had a bad case of it.

Dr.: Before Jessica was born?

Pt.: No, after she was born.

Dr.: After she was born. How old was she when the arthritis came?

Pt.: Oh, I would say (*pause*) a few months.

Dr.: A couple of months. Is that the first time you ever had arthritis?

Pt.: Yes, and it came as a sudden attack and the doctor thought it was rheumatic fever. He wasn't sure, and he took tests, and when he decided that it was rheumatoid arthritis, then the nerves took over.

Dr.: And you never had that before?

Pt.: No.

Dr.: So, at that time, ten years ago, you had a baby Jessica, named after you; and after she was born you had an attack of arthritis. How long did that last? (*What are felt to be important details in the history are repeated to the patient as a way of suggesting, impressing, and teaching the patient that this is important to her.*)

Pt.: I would say that lasted about two or three months.

Dr.: Have you had arthritis since?

Pt.: Well, I don't have severe pain with it. Sometimes my joints ache.

Dr.: Do you have swelling? (*A medical question asked to establish the severity of the condition.*)

Pt.: Just the fingers.

Dr.: Much?

Pt.: Like when the weather is bad they throb and they swell, and that's all.

Dr.: You are saying that you had arthritis after Jessica was born. You went to the movies, and you saw something medical and it was upsetting to you, and you don't think that you would have been upset if other things had been somewhat easier for you at that time. Then the arthritis went away.

Pt.: It seemed to.

Dr.: And then you say that the nerves took over?

Pt.: That's it.

Dr.: Do you remember in what way they took over?

Pt.: Most of the time it was heavy palpitations, and I never wanted to lay down because I could feel every pulse in my body pounding, and I would feel like I was going to faint all the time, and I didn't have any self confidence in going out. I never went out because I used to feel that I was going to pass out in the street.

Dr.: Did you look for help at that time?

Pt.: I went to several doctors, and they gave me different tranquilizers, and nothing seemed to work.

Dr.: You have been having this for ten years?

Pt.: Yes. Then I went to my obstetrician, and he gave me Doriden, and that seemed to help. I started to pick up a little bit. I used to rely on it, though. If I wanted to go out I would take Doriden, and I could go where I wanted to go and I could sleep. I couldn't sleep without it. But then, I had been on that quite a while.

Dr.: When you went to your obstetrician, were you pregnant at the time, or was it just that you go to him anyway?

Pt.: No, I wasn't pregnant. I was having so much trouble with the different tranquilizers that I just went to my obstetrician and told him how I felt, and he said that they seemed to be backfiring and that I needed something different. He gave me the Doriden.

Dr.: How long ago did you stop taking Doriden?

Pt.: I stopped taking it after I had the baby, before I had this last baby, which was nine months ago.

Dr.: So how long had you been taking Doriden?

Pt.: Seven years.

Dr.: How many times each day?

Pt.: I was taking three a day—well, not all the time. No, I would say for about four years I was taking three a day. The last few years I was taking half at a time to quiet me down during the day and then to sleep at night.

Dr.: When did you stop?

Pt.: When I got pregnant with this last baby, my doctor told me to stop. I stopped only when I got to the hospital. When I left the hospital I felt fine. She was born in February, and in April I had these terrific headaches so I went to the doctor.

Dr.: The same obstetrician?

Pt.: I changed obstetricians, and he thought that my pressure was up so he put me on something. Then the pains came back again, and he referred me to another—to a psychiatrist. (*The patient's long dependence on drugs is now apparent. Finally, she is referred to a psychiatrist.*)

Dr.: When did you see the psychiatrist?

Pt.: About four months ago, and he told me that the medication didn't help me. He said he would refer me here since I couldn't afford to go to him every week.

Dr.: And what did he give you?

Pt.: He have me Triavil and Librium, ten milligrams of each.

Dr.: How long did you continue to take these medicines?

Pt.: Until I came here about three weeks ago.

Dr.: Did it help you?

Pt.: No, I wasn't finding too much help from it. (*As it turns out, she has continued to take medication up to the day of this interview.*)

Dr.: Now then, in reviewing the information that you gave Dr. R. here, we hear that for at least ten years you have been nervous, anxious, frightened at times, and, as you put it, it seems as though after the arthritis the nerves took over. In all these years, have you any idea of your own as to what might be making you so nervous?

Pt.: No.

Dr.: No idea? (*Refuse to accept the immediate no.*)

Pt.: No, well, myself I don't know. I mean—people will tell me what they think is making me nervous, you know. Like the family will say that the children are making you nervous, or your childhood wasn't that happy and that is why you are nervous. But myself, I don't know why I am nervous.

Dr.: You have no idea yourself, and these ideas that other people tell you don't particularly strike you one way or another?

Pt.: No, well I figure that there are other people that have children, and they are not nervous, so why should mine make me nervous? (*She fixes on her children.*)

Dr.: How do you know that the other people aren't nervous? (*A mild effort to shake her sense of being uniquely nervous.*)

Pt.: Well, I see them going out every day, and some of them have ten children and they seem to be able to do what they want and go out.

Dr.: And you don't have ten—

Pt.: I have six.

Dr.: That's a healthy load.

Pt.: Active. (*She retranslates my term into one that is more meaningful to her.*)

Dr.: They keep you busy . . .

Pt.: They do.

Dr.: Alright, as I was saying, in reviewing the information that we have about you, it began ten years ago, and it seems to me that there are certain periods when it's gotten worse for you. (*A move to elaborate the repetition of her reactions and causes for them.*)

Pt.: During a crisis or anything I will feel worse.

Dr.: During a crisis you will feel worse—and which crises are you remembering?

Pt.: Well, my father's death.

Dr.: That was— (*Deliberate pause in order to let patient recall the time.*)

Pt.: Six years ago.

Dr.: What did he die of?

Pt.: A heart attack.

Dr.: Sudden?

Pt.: Yes. Well, he was only sick a few days, and we didn't expect—we just thought that he was going to get better.

Dr.: And you remember your reaction to that—to your father's death?

Pt.: Yes, I was very nervous—they had to give me an injection while I was in the hospital when he died.

Dr.: You were visiting?

Pt.: No, we took him to the hospital . . . While he was dying, we were waiting.

Dr.: They had to give you an injection because you were—

Pt.: So upset.

Dr.: Upset in what way?

Pt.: Well, I was shaky—I don't know, maybe that would be normal to anybody that was going through that.

Dr.: That was six years ago. Do you remember crying?

Pt.: Yes, I do.

Dr.: And then came the funeral—did you cry at the funeral?

Pt.: Oh, yes.

Dr.: Have you missed him since?

Pt.: Yes, I do.

Dr.: Think of him?

Pt.: I think of him all the time.

Dr.: All the time?

Pt.: I used to see a lot of him, and if I am alone my mind wanders and then I will think, and sometimes I think I wish he was here so that I could talk to him. Naturally, you like somebody to talk to, and when you have just the children around all the time— (*Grieved his loss but continues to mourn him.*)

Dr.: They are not much to talk to. (*She returns to the children as a burden.*)

Pt.: You get tired of the children—you don't of them, but you like to talk to adults after awhile.

Dr.: You do get tired of them, too, don't you?

Pt.: Well, I get tired of the demands that are made, but you try to fulfill them if you can.

Dr.: But you often think of your father?

Pt.: I do.

Dr.: And wish he were around to talk to? (*Back to the father in order to get more information about her reaction to his death.*)

Pt.: Yeah.

Dr.: Visit his grave?

Pt.: No.

Dr.: Ever?

Pt.: A couple of times I did.

Dr.: Do you ever cry about him now when you think of him?

Pt.: No.

Dr.: You don't. When your father died that was a crisis, and your nervousness got worse?

Pt.: For a while it did, yeah.

Dr.: Any other crisis?

Pt.: No, not that I can think of. Nothing that came up. But right now I have another because my mother is in the hospital.

Dr.: Wasn't there something, a crisis if you want to call it that, that came before your mother going to the hospital, when your symptoms got worse again?

Pt.: I don't know. I had pains in my head when I came here.

Dr.: Yes, but when you came here your mother wasn't in the hospital, and you didn't know she was going to be in the hospital.

Pt.: No.

Dr.: No, but you did say when you first came here that you were becoming increasingly nervous lately. What was the reason for this increase in your nervousness lately?

Pt.: I don't know. Of course, I was probably worried about my mother being alone because she lives alone.

Dr.: She has been living alone for quite some time.

Pt.: Since my father died.

Dr.: But why would your nervousness become worse in the past months, four, or five, or six months?

Pt.: I don't know.

Dr.: You did say that as I understand—

Pt.: I mentioned it.

Dr.: Should I remind you?

Pt.: No. Like I say, today, maybe my mind is in one place or another because I have just come from seeing my mother so I am a little upset.

Dr.: Well, what you had told us here was that since the birth of your newest baby—

Pt.: Oh, the new baby, Vivian.

Dr.: Yes, after Vivian's birth, you began to—

Pt.: It was just four months later, and the doctor said that he thought it was just the delayed—like some get the blues right after their birth and I never did. As a matter of fact, nobody would understand, being such a nervous person, how I could go home from the hospital and be so happy.

Dr.: You didn't get nervous?

Pt.: No. But he thought maybe just a delayed reaction.

Dr.: Four months after her birth you started—

Pt.: I started—

Dr.: What did you feel?

Pt.: I was getting these pains going up the back of my head, and I didn't know what that was.

Dr.: Anything else?

Pt.: And I wasn't taking any medication at the time. I had gotten off the Doriden, and what I was doing was that I was having one or two beers at night, and that would help me to sleep. I was taking care of the children and going out, and I felt fine. And then all of a sudden, I got that pain, and it kind of scared me.

Dr.: Was there anything else that you felt? How about your nervous symptoms?

Pt.: I was nervous and I was anxious, and when I went to the doctor he knew then.

Dr.: When you say that you were anxious, what do you mean?

Pt.: The only way that I can seem to describe how I feel inside my head is as if I had seen an awful accident. My insides are all trembling. When I get like that I can't seem to control it. I sit down and try to quiet myself down—(*Frightened about seeing someone get hurt.*)

Dr.: Well, that's a very keen way of describing the way you feel—anxious as though you were seeing someone—

Pt.: As though I were seeing—like any normal—like anybody would see an accident and get very upset. And I get like that for nothing.

Dr.: Did you say automobile accident? (*She hadn't. This was my own association in thinking about her family of six living in an urban area.*)

Pt.: Any kind of an accident—anything that you would see that would upset you. I can imagine anybody walking on the street that saw any kind of accident would get emotional.

Dr.: There are all kinds of accidents.

Pt.: I suppose.

Dr.: What kind of accident do you think of that frightens you?

Pt.: Well, I mean if I were seeing somebody—like a car accident. I mean, I have seen several cars collide and I start shaking—you know, thinking something like maybe somebody got hurt—that's the effect.

Dr.: Have you ever seen anyone get hurt in an accident?

Pt.: No. (*We get some pointed information about her fears of her own aggression concealed within her nervousness.*)

Dr.: The anxiousness is something like an accident happening, or somebody gets hurt and you don't want to see it. It began ten years ago—it became worse, perhaps the way you described it, when your father died, and you reacted again after the birth of your last child, and very recently with the illness of your mother. What's the matter with her? (*I repeat, for emphasis, the last three crises.*)

Pt.: Well, she was operated on yesterday for cancer of her bowels.

Dr.: Something unexpected?

Pt.: Yes, I just brought her into the hospital a week ago last Saturday. She had pains in her stomach and I brought her in.

Dr.: Who is responsible for her—for looking after her? I know you have a doctor but who is responsible in the family? (*Investigating her evident distress now that even more responsibility is imposed upon her.*)

Pt.: I handle all her personal affairs.

Dr.: You do?

Pt.: Yes.

Dr.: What has been your reaction to her illness now?

Pt.: I wasn't very optimistic—I gave in and figured at her age I didn't think they could do much for her. The operation has been a success, but they don't know whether she'll pull through. But they say she is doing well, so I am accepting that.

Dr.: Have you been nervous since you took her to the hospital?

Pt.: Well, I realize that I wasn't able to go a couple of times to see her. (*Her fear of going out.*)

Dr.: And isn't it since you took your mother to the hospital that a rash began?

Pt.: Yes. It started out in big welts, and I suppose all the scratching made it like this (*as she shows her arm*), like it was hives, and now it's all welts all over my body.

Dr.: Have you ever had that before?

Pt.: No.

Dr.: Never?

Pt.: Never. I have psoriasis.

Dr.: You do have psoriasis? Any now?

Pt.: Yes it is on my body.

Dr.: How long have you had psoriasis?

Pt.: I have had it since about sixteen or seventeen.

Dr.: But never hives?

Pt.: No, never.

Dr.: How much trouble does the psoriasis give you?

Pt.: It doesn't bother me too often—maybe once or twice a year where it has a point where it gets a little itchy, but it's not too bad.

Dr.: But you have it almost all the time.

Pt.: Yeah.

Dr.: Do you ever have it in places that are exposed?

Pt.: I have it sometimes on my arms and legs, but if I can get out in the sun it helps.

Dr.: Anyone else in your family with psoriasis?

Pt.: No—just me.

Dr.: You never had hives before. How long ago is it that it broke out?

Pt.: I would say—today is Friday—last Thursday.

Dr.: What do you think did it?

Pt.: Well—when I brought my mother to the hospital, when she had to have a certain kind of test done—she didn't want it done, and she kind of scared me. She said she wanted to go home, and I wasn't about to go through all that and just let her go home because I knew what was the matter, and I think that kind of gave me a jolt. I tried to hold in what I knew and didn't want to tell her because it would upset her.

Dr.: She didn't want the test done, and she wanted you to take her home.

Pt.: I refused and I walked away. After that I seemed to hold back because I knew what was wrong, and I couldn't tell her. (*To "hold back" is typical of her, and the many physical symptoms fail, nevertheless, to contain her anxiety.*)

Dr.: When, then, did the hives appear?

Pt.: The next day.

Dr.: The next day you had the hives. Have you been scratching ever since?

Pt.: Yes, I tried Benadryl but it made me sick—and yet the doctor said it shouldn't have.

Dr.: What I would like to do now is to see how we could get at what might be the most important thing that is troubling you. When I asked you what it is that you would most want help with, what did you say?

Pt.: Well—so that I could take care of my children. I would like to feel normal. I would like to be able to get up in the morning and send my family off to school and work and take care of the two little ones and not have this anxiety—not be afraid to be left alone. (*This time she links her anxiety with the burden of her children and being left alone.*)

Dr.: And not be afraid that something might happen or that you might see something terrible?

Pt.: My main fear is that when I get these feelings—if I pass out and the two little ones are alone, what would happen?

Dr.: It seems to me, and you know this yourself, this isn't new—it has been going on for ten years. Ten years is when you had the arthritis, and ten years is when you went to the movie, and ten years is when your daughter, Jessica, was born—all starting at that time. Now, the way that I would look at it is this: I think that the thing that bothers you—and I am going to put it in a very general sense until we can make it even clearer—but I think that the thing that most bothers you is that you have a nagging sense of discontent, of irritability, and of tension. Does that sound familiar? Or will you just say yes because you think that you should? (*I review and re-translate what she means about her children; I emphasize the long history and present her with a central issue.*)

Pt.: Irritable about what?

Dr.: That remains to be found out.

Pt.: Discontent?

Dr.: Discontent—nagging sense of discontent. Do you know what I mean by that?

Pt.: Do you mean like the same routine? (*She sharpens the central issue.*)

Dr.: That would be one of the things that would certainly contribute to it. By nagging sense, I mean a kind of vague feeling—you are just not pleased with the way your life is going even though you may not put your finger exactly—

Pt.: On it.

Dr.: On it. And with such a nagging sense of discontent anyone would be irritable, or more easily irritated, than you ordinarily are. I would say that we have to find out as much as we can about the major problem of discontent. Does that strike a reasonable note for you, or do you think of something else?

Pt.: No.

Dr.: Does this seem like something that might be useful to you if we were to look at this idea?

Pt.: Mmmmmm.

Dr.: Because I know that you are discontented. (*A direct diagnostic statement that is not a guess but born out of the data.*)

Pt.: Well—I will go as far as saying that I am very unhappy. I mean, there isn't anything to look forward to if you think you're going to go through the same thing day after day. Like the way I feel, I have six healthy children that I would like to be able to enjoy them—and a good husband, and it doesn't seem fair to them.

Dr.: But you are not happy.

Pt.: No. I am happy when I have them all together.

Dr.: I think that you are saying that you are happy *for them* but *you* are not happy—

Pt.: For myself—

Dr.: What I would like to suggest is this—this is where you and I will direct our attention—to the fact that you are discontented and even unhappy, and see if we can figure out what this is all about. We will spend all our time on that and more than that. I will see you each week at 1:15 right here—I want to make it very clear—each Friday, from 1:15 to 2:00. Is that a good time for you?

Pt.: That will be alright for me.

Dr.: I am going to see you twelve times including today, and those twelve times will end on Friday, January thirty-first. I will not be here on January third so I will have to skip that one. If we go along without you missing any appointments and without my missing except for January third, we will finish the twelve appointments on Friday, January thirty-first. If anything comes up, like snowstorms, we will manage that as they come along. However, as it stands, I will see you each Friday, 1:15 to 2:00, twelve times, and during those twelve times we will try to work as much as we can on this problem of your general discontent. If, in the course of our discussions it turns out that there is something else that is even more important, we will go into that. What do you think about the idea?

Pt.: Alright—that seems alright to me. (*Arthritis, phobias, anxiety attacks, psoriasis, hives, depression, gastrointestinal distress. These indicate not only widespread causality but, more important, in the interview they tell us that they are used to conceal, to keep out of awareness, active response or responses to intolerable relationships with her environment and the people in it. A broad, nonspecific focus is offered which is diagnostic, expresses the final common pathway of the complicated, multicausal, unconsciously motivated symptoms, and allows the patient an entrée into her difficulties which she not only understands but feels.*)

Dr.: Do you have any question about it?

Pt.: No. The only question is about medication. Do I still stay on the Librium?

Dr.: How much and how often are you taking it?

Pt.: Twenty-five milligrams three times a day.

Dr.: What do you think would happen it you didn't take it?

Pt.: Then I have these anxious feelings.

Dr.: How do you know that you will have these anxious feelings if you don't take it. When did you start the Librium?

Pt.: Started in June (*about four months ago*).

Dr.: Every day since then?

Pt.: I was taking ten milligrams until I came here and the doctor gave me twenty-five.

Dr.: What do you think will happen if you stopped all medication between now and next Friday?

Pt.: Well, I know I would get that way. Like my husband says, "If you stop and you get that way, maybe you will get over it." He seems to think that I don't give a fair chance—

Dr.: That you don't give what?

Pt.: Like the medication—I seem to rely on it as a crutch.

Dr.: Maybe you are somewhat afraid not to take it.

Pt.: I am. I am afraid that I won't be able to take care of things.

Dr.: I would not be at all surprised that you would be able to take care of things without needing all those crutches now . . . Suppose that you didn't take any medicine until I see you next Friday. (*Pressing her to rely on herself.*) Do you think that you can manage that?

Pt.: I will give it a try, but supposing—

Dr.: Supposing—than you know what to do. (*She is free to take medication or not.*)

Pt.: Take them.

Dr.: Unless you feel that you can do without them.

Pt.: I am willing to give it a try because I didn't think that I could get off Doriden and I did.

Dr.: And some of these things are better not taken too long. Is my proposal clear to you—that we will meet each week?

Pt.: Each week and discuss my discontentment and unhappiness.

Dr.: Discontentment and unhappiness, and we will stick with that barring interruptions that we can't foresee. Then you and I will be finished with this work on the thirty-first of January.

Pt.: Do you think I will be alright—I mean, I don't know if I am being presumptuous asking you.

Dr.: You can ask anything.

Pt.: Do you think that you can help me? If you do then I am willing to try to go without the medication and see what happens.

Dr.: Yes.

Pt.: Okay, if you think you can help me, then I can stop the pills. (*I repeat the treatment plan, and she finally can ask me directly whether it will help. My positive response leads her to do likewise.*)

Dr.: We still have some time left today so we can go further on this question of your unhappiness. (*Immediate return to the central issue.*)

Pt.: I am not unhappy with my immediate family, my husband or my children. I was unhappy with my mother. I tried to take over when my father died—

Dr.: to do all I could, and she was a dominant person, and that had a lot to do with it. She would interfere. . . .

Dr.: You say that one of the things that gets at you is that every day you know exactly what tomorrow is going to be. It's going to be like today. (*I preferred to keep her very much alive feelings about her present situation in the forefront rather than go back in time at this point.*)

Pt.: That's right—until my mother went into the hospital, every day was a ritual. I had to get up and get on the telephone, and I had to call her and see how she was. In the meantime, my four-year-old would be tearing the house apart, and by the time I got through with that I would be ready to tear the roof down. I didn't want to scream over the telephone, but I knew what every day would bring because now she's in the hospital—I don't have the phone calls, but I've so many other things to occupy my mind—I don't see any difference. (*"Tear the roof down" in her anger, which, as we see, is not relieved by the temporary lessening of demands by her mother.*)

Dr.: Every day is still the same.

Pt.: Still the same. .

Dr.: Well, you have six kids.

Pt.: That's what people can't understand. How can I get so bored or upset with having the children around.

Dr.: People really don't understand that six kids could tie a woman down with the same thing every day. They don't understand that. I bet you would like a vacation.

Pt.: I would. We took one once, and we are still paying for it—two or three years ago. I said to my husband that I couldn't take it anymore and I would like a trip. We took a trip to Washington with all five children.

Dr.: Do you ever get a day off by yourself without any of the children?

Pt.: No. I never bothered. I can if I want to—my husband is willing. He takes them on the weekend, and sometimes I feel, well, why is he taking them and leaving me behind and alone? He will take them off my hands to let me lay down or rest, but I don't seem to want to do that. Then if he suggests to get a babysitter and go out I feel nervous, and I don't want to go out. (*A characteristic neurotic expression of the angry wish and the defense against it. She would love to be free but the wish is so loaded with anger and guilt as to block the opportunity for its fulfillment.*)

Dr.: When your husband does offer to get a babysitter, you don't want to go out?

Pt.: I'm nervous when I go out, and I wish I weren't out, and I worry about the children—if they are alright and—

Dr.: You are really tied down aren't you?

Pt.: I am tied to my children too much probably. Like I always was, I used to have a fear of death. The doctor said that even when I am gone they will live, so why do I worry about it.

Dr.: Is it that you have a fear of dying, or is it that you fear what will happen to the children?

Pt.: It's mostly the children.

Dr.: You are not so much afraid that you might die?

Pt.: No, only when I get these pains in my head. Sometimes I get pressure and I feel as if my head is going to burst. I feel like I have something there. My husband helps to quiet me down.

Dr.: Does the fact of dying frighten you personally, apart from the children?

Pt.: I shouldn't be frightened. We all have to go.

Dr.: Yes, but most people are afraid of dying.

Pt.: I think that I never was like that until my father died. Ever since then any pains I have had I always thought I was having a heart attack like my father.

Dr.: Well, I gather that you are very much tied down to your house and that even the offer to go out for an evening is not a very attractive one for you—it's even a scary one—so you stay in the house.

Pt.: I do. I try to take the baby out, but I don't venture too far from the house. I stay close. I have friends that meet once a week, but then I got tired of going to that because I was listening to all their problems—they were having trouble with their husbands—they thought I was odd because I got along with my husband, so I stopped that. I have my own problems and I have a good husband, so there wasn't any point into looking into somebody else's—probably try to put something into your mind, you know.

Dr.: But things go on in everyday work in the house, so that after awhile you feel you are ready to tear the roof—

Pt.: I get so that sometimes I just don't want to prepare the meals even. I get tired. Of course, sometimes I even feel that if I had a demanding husband I wouldn't be the way that I am.

Dr.: How do you mean that?

Pt.: I will say that most of the time I have gotten dinner prepared because he has to hurry and he only has a half hour to eat and get off to school. Then he will turn around and say, "If you don't feel like doing anything, a sandwich is fine"—and I will say, "Oh, no, not after working all day." The housework—he says, "Leave it. If you don't want to do it, don't do it." I figure if maybe he says sometimes, "Do this and do that," maybe I would do it.

Dr.: Think it would help sometimes if he gave you a swat?

Pt.: Once a doctor told him not to sympathize with me. (*If her husband were less passive and more demanding, she would feel relieved somewhat of her guilt and at the same time would be able to feel more justified in her anger—a demand for a more adaptive kind of sadomasochistic relationship.*) I used to wake him up at three in the morning when I had these feelings, and naturally he was tired; he would have to get up for work. The doctor told him to argue with me, so then he would start at me, and then I would get angry, and I would go to sleep and the feeling was gone.

Dr.: What was there about that that made you angry?

Pt.: Because he didn't think that I was sick.

Dr.: He wasn't taking seriously the fear that you would die?

Pt.: Yes. But I found out he was more concerned than I realized. But I have no one to argue with during the day. The two babies can't argue with me, and then I try to fight it myself, you know.

Dr.: But, that example that you gave of your husband in the middle of the night—you would feel better if you got a little bit off your—

Pt.: Chest.

Dr.: Chest. I would gather that is one aspect of your unhappiness. I mentioned to you earlier that I think that you also suffer from easy irritability, easily irritated—

Pt.: I can be easily irritated.

Dr.: This suggests that part of your unhappiness is because you are angry about something or some things. (*I refine the focus a bit more.*)

Pt.: Probably take it out on somebody else.

Dr.: I know who you take it out on.

Pt.: Myself.

Dr.: Yes.

Pt.: I don't know. Sometimes if I wonder—several doctors have asked how is your married life—if I don't have something to complain about when I get along so good, why should things be like this?

Dr.: Sometimes there are things that bother us and we are really not aware of what they are. They are somewhere inside us. We don't know what they are, and we need help to find out what they are. (*Supportive education.*)

Pt.: I think if the shoe were on the other foot, I don't know if I could have stood anybody as long as he has had to stand me and put up with it. In a way, there can't be too much wrong with me. I have had three more children since all of this happened.

Dr.: You do your own housework.

Pt.: Of course, I have an older daughter and she helps.

Dr.: And you keep your house going.

Pt.: I try.

Dr.: Ever fall flat on your face?

Pt.: Some days I just sit down and I don't want to do it. It's not that I can't, I don't want to. I haven't any incentive.

Dr.: What happens that day—just sit?

Pt.: No, you can't just sit. You have to do the laundry if there are babies—but I feel there is no point in doing the work because the children just upset it, and I just get discouraged, and I don't bother. Then my husband comes home and says, "So what? Clean it later." Or he will say, "Let's do it together."

Dr.: So he comes home and you are discouraged all day—haven't done a thing that you know you should have been doing. You tell him and he says that's alright, so you don't do it. How do you react to that when he says that?

Pt.: I always figure that if it was somebody else, they would have something else to say.

Dr.: Yeah, give you a boot and say, "Come on let's get going."

Pt.: Do something.

Dr.: Then you can't get mad at him.

Pt.: Yeah.

Dr.: I suppose that is is hard to get mad at someone who doesn't fight.

Pt.: The only arguments that we have are over the children. I said to him, "I don't know, maybe I would feel better if we had more arguments."

Dr.: What does he say to that?

Pt.: "What are we going to argue over?"

Dr.: Our time is up today. We'll continue on this next Friday at 1:15.

My opening question immediately directed the patient's attention to a central issue. From this point on, I sought information about her present complaints, similar or related complaints from the past, and other factual information. She appears to have a host of psychophysiological symptoms and reveals herself to be a conscientious, compulsive (albeit warm and sweet in demeanor) woman who cannot allow herself recognition that the burden she feels she endures is often too much for her. It must have always been so for her. That is, her adaptive style was not arrived at only since she became a mother and housewife. The focus presented is deliberately made broad and inclusive but covers, in fact, exactly what she is feeling and cannot let herself know. Note that the global central issue is almost immediately made more precise in the patient's swift rejoinder that she "will go as far as saying that I am very unhappy."

This first interview has been presented almost in its entirety, since it illustrates so well the procedure for creating the kind of structure that will influence the flow of the treatment process.

Second Interview

She begins by telling me that things are better. Her rash has improved, and she has stopped taking her previous medication: "I did what you asked me to do last time." She told her husband that I had said that she is unhappy, and he accepted that. Having reported these gains, she then introduces a new symptom.

Pt.: I can't eat. I can't seem to eat. I feel nauseated all the time. My stomach is jumping all the time and I can't eat.

Dr.: Is this something different for you, not to be eating?

Pt.: Mmmm. I put on thirty-eight pounds after I had the baby from eating too much. This is new.

Dr.: It started last week?

Pt.: It started when I stopped taking the medication.

Dr.: And that was last week. When did you stop eating? . . .

Pt.: Let's see. Well, I didn't eat when I went home Friday.

Dr.: Is that when it began?

Pt.: As far as I can remember back. Like Friday, I didn't have much of an appetite at suppertime, and then Saturday I didn't feel like eating. Like I say, I try to force myself when my husband is around. He says if you don't eat you are not going to get better either.

Dr.: Would you say that?

Pt.: Of course—I have a cold, too. A bad cold. (A profusion of symptoms to keep both of us in the dark as to their source.)

Dr.: But this is all something different for you because you've been eating a lot.

Pt.: I have.

Dr.: Last Friday, very suddenly, you stopped.

Pt.: No, I wouldn't say suddenly. I had the food in front of me, and I just felt nauseous.

Dr.: Beginning last Friday.

Pt.: Last week.

Dr.: Last Friday. Is that right or am I wrong?

Pt.: No. Last Friday after I left here. I was a little nervous, and I was anticipating being off the pills. I cross my bridges way ahead of them, and I kept thinking that I am going to be alone with the children and kept getting jumpy . . .

Dr.: It is possible that the nausea and the lack of appetite have to do with the fact that you have not been taking the pills, which is the first time in a long time.

Pt.: Yes. But see, it didn't happen when I had the baby and I stopped taking my Doriden. I kept on eating like I was eating in the hospital plus adding more, and I was taking too good care of myself and put all the weight on. (*This discussion of her loss of appetite is cautiously investigative. The symptom began very promptly after her first treatment interview. It is possible that she was suffering the side effects of the medication for her hives, very likely antihistamines. However, the dramatic suddenness of the symptom and its intensity in a woman who has been overeating give one pause as to its psychological significance. I chose to understand the symptom as a reaction to the oral sadism unleashed when she agreed to stop taking pills and could anticipate oral fulfillment in the treatment plan that she accepted. The danger of being overwhelmed with devouring fantasies is prevented by the appearance of anorexia and nausea. It would not be wise to tamper with her defenses around such sensitive fantasies and fears in this kind of short treatment, and I decided to leave it.*)

Dr.: Anything else beside the nausea and no appetite?

Pt.: No.

Dr.: Are you sleeping well? (*In the light of all previous information, including her stopping the pills, I could assume that she was not sleeping well.*)

Pt.: No. I have to lay there and watch television until my eyes close or until there isn't any more television left to watch.

Dr.: So this past week it's been nausea, and not eating well, and having trouble sleeping.

Pt.: Not as much trouble as I had years ago. At least this past week I have gone to bed knowing what to expect.

Dr.: What else this week?

Pt.: Well, I went out yesterday. It was the first time that I went out without medication or anything, and I felt that I had done something. I had to go to school for the children.

Dr.: You went out alone?

Pt.: Yeah.

Dr.: Without medication. You should be proud of yourself.

Pt.: That's what my husband said. I said you would think that I was one of the children in school. (*An interesting mixture of being proud of her adult accomplishment and yet feeling the childishness in making much of the accomplishment.*)

Dr.: Still, it's not easy.

Pt.: No, it wasn't easy, but it was worth going out. I got good reports from the school and that made me feel good, too. Then I came home, and I went out again. I went shopping.

Dr.: Alone?

Pt.: Alone? No. I took two of the little ones with me, which I never like to do—

Dr.: Because—

Pt.: I always feel that if I get sick or something, the children are left alone. That's why I don't like to take the baby out. (*The fear of her unconscious wish to abandon the little ones and be relieved of responsibility for them.*)

Dr.: What happened?

Pt.: What happened? Nothing.

Dr.: (*Affirmatively.*) Nothing.

Pt.: No, it's awful hard to face. You know that it's there, and yet to overcome it.

Dr.: Your good sense tells you that nothing is there but nevertheless you *feel* differently.

Pt.: If I could only conquer that—you know—jumpy feeling. I feel as if I am sitting on a bomb and it's going to explode at any time. I always feel as though something is going to be wrong. (*"Tear the roof off" and now "sitting on a bomb," along with the pains in her head that sometimes threaten to burst her head open, speak eloquently to the enormous rage that she struggles to control through her manifold symptoms and characterological defenses.*)

Dr.: You feel like you are sitting on a bomb?

Pt.: I feel something . . . something is going to go wrong. Instead of just keeping my mind blank and going on with my work, I keep my mind going instead of just busying myself.

Dr.: How do you mean, mind going?

Pt.: Instead of just doing my work, I will be thinking of the children coming home, and all the excitement, and getting dinner ready, and things like that.

Dr.: You find yourself thinking of all the things that you will have to do.

Pt.: If I know that something is coming up six months from now, I will start worrying about it today. (*The anxious anticipation of responsibility means the constant presence of time as a ruling factor in her life—and she knows when treatment will end.*)

Dr.: You are always thinking of what next you have to do?

Pt.: That's right.

Dr.: It must make you feel overloaded.

Pt.: I feel like I want to take the knapsack off my back and drop it. But it really isn't that much of a load. I don't know why it should be bothering me. (*Always a load on her back that she would like to be rid of—followed by quick denial.*)

Dr.: Well, may be it is a load . . . (*She continues with a description of herself as a perfectionist, always thinking ahead of what has to be done so that she constantly feels burdened, tense, and uncertain whether she can cope with it all. She cannot tolerate disorder or her failure to perform. The combination makes her feel that she is always sitting on a bomb. She knows that it is not possible to keep up with every detail of work and to manage six children, but she feels compelled to do so, nevertheless. She then compares her own family-size history with that of her mother. Mother had ten pregnancies and lost five in miscarriages; the patient has had eight pregnancies and has lost two in miscarriages.*)

Pt.: I did alright until the fourth came, and then I began slowing down. But the Doriden helped me along so I was able to do everything.

Dr.: Are you saying that things changed in a way after Jessica was born?

Pt.: A year after.

Dr.: That would be the ten years. Tell me about Jessica.

Pt.: I think she sees too much of my nerves—She is getting to be a nervous child. (*To hear about Jessica is to hear about the patient.*)

Dr.: Really?

Pt.: She seems to have a lot of aches and pains. I brought her to the hospital, and there is nothing there. I keep saying to my husband, I think that she is watching me too much. She is the last of the older ones to leave in the morning. She will ask me if I am alright. . . . If I say no, she will say, "Well, I don't feel good; I will stay home." As bad as I feel, I say, "No, you go to school." Sometimes she will stay home, and as schooltime starts she is alright, so then I figure there's nothing wrong. I hope that I am just not passing what's in me off to her. (*Jessica exhibits signs of a mild phobic attachment ot her mother. Note the intuitive awareness of this unsophisticated woman in respect to the unhealthy identification of each with the other. If the patient is helped in her treatment, we may be assured that the daughter will profit equally.*)

Dr.: Tell me more about Jessica. What kind of a kid is she?

Pt.: She's a good little kid. She doesn't get into any trouble in school or anything. She's in the middle and gets pushed around by her brothers and sisters, but other than that she's good and she plays well. . . . I mean, she has her friends and she goes out . . . (*So, too, is the patient a "good little kid." She goes on to describe further her relationship with Jessica. Jessica not only obeys like her mother, but also whines and cries a good deal. The patient cannot tolerate this and frequently slaps her with the excuse that she must learn not to cry for nothing. As a result, Jessica is struck more than any of the children, and the patient thinks that this is Jessica's way of seeking attention. Their relationship is a beautiful example of a child becoming the projected image of the mother's wishes and feelings about herself—wishes and feelings that must be denied within herself.*)

Dr.: So pretty much most of your life is taken up by this thing—which one is in trouble, and which one is fussing, and which one is crying, and which one is hollering, misbehaving. (*I emphasize the ever present pressures on her and my understanding of what she must endure.*)

Pt.: And they're not doing—not doing well in school. One won't do his homework, and the other one stayed up last night until 12:30 with homework.

Dr.: I gather that you are the kind of person who really feels best if everything is really clicking and going along the way you want it to—the house clean and in order, the children neat and taking care of things and doing what they're supposed to do and doing alright in school, not getting in trouble— (*Acknowledging what she knows herself to be.*)

Pt.: Then I figure there would be harmony that way. You can't have it being at one another's throat.

Dr.: But see this, too, that beginning ten years ago when Jessica came along— It was at that point that you felt that you were no longer able to keep things together or to keep up things the way you always did. You have always had this need to keep up and stay ahead.

Pt.: Yeah, I have always wanted to you know—just so.

Dr.: You are a very conscientious person. (*This remark must reverberate in her unconscious because it rewards her demanding superego but must also remind her of her unacceptable wishes and the deeply felt guilt about them.*)

Pt.: Actually, I am.

Dr.: I *know* you are.

Pt.: I know it can't be done, and yet I can't make myself understand it can't be done. For the house to be just so, the children would just have to be sitting all the time, which doesn't make sense either. . . (*Here she elaborates on her compulsive need to have her house in order. She fears having someone come into her home and find it untidy. It is important that others see her house, which represents the patient, as tidy, orderly, and clean and not upset or bad. She becomes discouraged and depressed when she finds it impossible to maintain her required standards of order. She fights the battle between order and disorder, and this is followed by a helpless depression which becomes lightened only with the magical hope that somehow all will be once more well.*)

Pt.: When I am not feeling good it doesn't bother me. When I have that spark of energy in me, and I just open my eyes and I can see everything that needs to be done, then I start. So, I am better off to stay sick. Then I can't see it.

Dr.: You stay sick—what do you mean?

Pt.: If I am nervous or anything, I couldn't care less how upset the house was. (*The secondary gain of illness.*)

Dr.: At that point you don't care. So you are better off if you stay nervous. (*Challenge her neurotic gain.*)

Pt.: No, well actually I am not. But then there would be times when I would go out and come back and sometimes my daughter will have the house all picked up. Maybe she'll have one of the children in bed, and it will be all nice and clean and it makes me feel good.

Dr.: You have always been this way, haven't you?

Pt.: As far as I can remember. It was always the same way at home. Everything had to be kept in order and that's how my mother kept house. But she did it with everybody helping her.

Dr.: I bet you helped.

Pt.: I did my share . . . I had to do my share, you know, because I was left. I was the last one left so I had the whole thing at the end before I got married. (*Again the denial of excessive demand on her, followed by confirmation that that is exactly what happened.*)

Dr.: And you did it.

Pt.: Yeah, I did it.

Dr.: You were a good kid.

Pt.: That's how I was brought up. I was to do that.

Dr.: Weren't you the best one?

Pt.: Well, I think that I was.

Dr.: I bet you were. You helped your mother and did what she asked you to do. She was strict about this kind of thing.

Pt.: It had to be done. We could have time once the work was done—once your work was done.

Dr.: And you obeyed.

Pt.: I did, yeah.

Dr.: Did you ever, say, rebel and refuse?

Pt.: The only time I ever rebelled was when my father died and she came to live with me. I was pregnant, and I just couldn't take any more. (*Cannot recall rebelling until age thirty-three for the first time.*)

Dr.: And that was just six years ago.

Pt.: We still do what my mother tells us. I still jump through the hoop.

Dr.: How do you feel about that?

Pt.: Like I said time and time again, I am married, and I have my family, and I should be my own boss, and I don't need anybody telling me how to do things, you know. Sometimes I think that's why I am so conscious—conscientious about the house and things. Because my mother would be there and she would be saying this should be done and that should be done—and I would be running around with the children trying to do for them and I would be listening to her—and you know, I think that's where I got like that instead of accepting an upset house. (*Mother is always with her in her mind.*)

Dr.: In other words, even to this day, you always have in back of your mind what would happen if your mother walked in.

Pt.: That's right. I don't have it in my mind; it's in my mouth constantly.

Dr.: You mean—

Pt.: Pick it up. If your grandmother ever walked in she would die. So then they have to start jumping and picking up if they know that she's coming. It's about the only time they will jump because they don't want to listen to her—because then she will start on them. (*"Speck of dust and see mother bust."*)

Dr.: She will get after them?

Pt.: You are making your mother sick, she would say to them. I would tell her it's not my children, it's from a long time ago, and she wouldn't accept it.

Dr.: Were you looking at her when you told her that?

Pt.: Oh yes—and she wouldn't accept it, and I said, "Well, I am sorry, but that's how it was put to me—that it didn't start with my marriage and my children—that I had a nervous bringing up when I was small." I wasn't happy in that house.

Dr.: That you had a nervous bringing up?

Pt.: I was very nervous when I was children—when I was a child. Gosh, talking about my children. (*Her identification with her own children as a needing person.*)

Dr.: How do you mean that you were a very nervous child?

Pt.: Well, the house wasn't happy. My father used to drink and come in and start arguing. I would be looking for that every night when he would go out the door. I would be sitting there anticipating what would be coming when he would come home. That's where I probably learned this business of looking forward all the time . . . (*Her experience with mother and father tells us something about her own tendency always to be looking ahead expecting something bad to happen—a very fine bit of insight on her part. Note here one of the meanings of time for this patient: the constant looking ahead, waiting for a dreaded event to occur. She describes her father as becoming rambunctious at times and clarifies her own fears of aggression as a result of her witnessing gross aggression between her parents. In later years, father quieted down. Nevertheless, she tells of her conviction*

*that her nervousness began with these repeated frightening scenes at home,
so that she knew herself to be a frightened child. Thus, she felt herself
trapped between a demanding mother and a father who would so terrify
her.)*

Dr.: How did it turn out?

Pt.: To be sick like this and nervous for almost nothing.

Dr.: Oh, it's not for nothing—you have your reasons. We were talking about it
last week. You are unhappy and discontented about something. (*As she
seeks to dispose of the present distress by simply attaching it to the past
and letting it go at that, I remind her of the central issue.*)

Pt.: Well, about all that I could think of that would make me unhappy now is
the house.

Dr.: Which house are you talking about?

Pt.: My house, presently.

Dr.: Yes. On the other hand, you were telling me that when you were a little
girl you learned to behave. Your mother taught you what she wanted you
to do, and you do it to this day. (*Clarifying and relating past and present
behavior in the "house."*)

Pt.: Still do it.

Dr.: You are afraid of her. You were afraid of your father, too.

Pt.: In a different sense, in a different way.

Dr.: Different way—when he came home that way. How was it between you
and him otherwise when you were a kid?

Pt.: He was a likeable person.

Dr.: When he wasn't drinking.

Pt.: He never yelled or hit us, you know. I never remember having gotten a
licking in my life, which is unusual. I must have been as bad as other children at some time or other.

Dr.: But weren't you a very good girl?

Pt.: It seems impossible that I wouldn't have to have a licking. I must have had
one somewhere.

Dr.: You don't remember—

Pt.: I don't remember—

Dr.: Because you were a very good kid. And I am not saying that sarcastically.

Pt.: I was good because I had to be . . . Maybe I didn't want to be.

Dr.: That's right.

Pt.: But I didn't dare be otherwise, so that's why I probably didn't get the
lickings, because I was smart enough to be good—do what I was told . . .
(*"I had to be good"—fear was the moving force in promoting an adaptive
mode. To overcome fear and anger meant to avoid them by giving no
reason for others to become antagonistic toward her. Much of her anxiety
and its attendant symptoms arises directly from her unconscious wish to be
"bad." She fears badness out of her experiences with her parents' capacity
for aggression and her fantasies about her own badness and aggression—the
bomb within her, for example. The patient then goes on to say that she is
no longer afraid of her mother, but rather it is out of respect for her that
she will not oppose her. She feels that she is like her mother in some ways
and watches herself with her own children because "I don't want them to
do what I want because they are afraid of me." She has told her daughter
that she hopes that when the girl is married, she will be able to tell her*

SECOND INTERVIEW109

mother to mind her own business if she is interfering. She wants this be-
cause "there isn't any happiness there if you have to be forever listening
when you don't want to." She finds herself looking about the house and
wondering what would happen if her mother walked in—always listening
to her and for her. She is unable to behave in any way other than to do
what she is told to do. I follow on this with a supportive enumeration of
the heavy burdens that she bears, laced with repeated remarks suggesting
her feelings about all this. Thus, I tell her that I can understand what she
feels as a person who always carries a heavy sense of responsibility, one
who must do what she feels she is supposed to do, how she always hears
her mother tell her to do and is afraid to say no, that she has six children
and how difficult it is to keep everything in order in the face of misbehav-
ing children, and how upsetting this is for her as the kind of person who
needs everything to go right.)

Pt.: Mmmmm. I would like it to be smooth all the time.

Dr.: Well, I think that everybody would. But you have a greater need for things
to be neat and clean and go well, and when they don't—and with six kids
it's very hard—it gets you, and it makes you nervous.

Pt.: It does. And then I end up, not taking it out on them. I take it out on
myself. I keep it inside.

Dr.: Keep what inside?

Pt.: Instead of yelling about anything, I will hold it in.

Dr.: Alright, then you are saying it makes you nervous, and it really makes you
angry. You are pretty damned mad at them, aren't you?

Pt.: I am, and I get tired of speaking to them, so then I just hold it in.

Dr.: Are you aware that you are—have a lot of anger in you, and you don't
know what to do with it?

Pt.: Oh yes, I can see myself getting, you know, mad at times. I used to holler
a lot but I got tired of that. I wasn't getting anywhere with it. I tried speaking with them but they are deaf. They don't want to listen.

Dr.: And that, of course, upsets you still more.

Pt.: I get a little irritated with it. I will accept more with the little ones. The
older ones should know better but they don't. I mean, they are babies in a
way. You know you can't put old heads on young shoulders . . . (*Denial is
in operation again.*)

Dr.: You are the kind of person who always feels that you have to please, don't
you?

Pt.: I do.

Dr.: Are you saying that to please me?

Pt.: No. I feel guilty sometimes. Sometimes I would like to—I would try to
please a person when I would like to tell them to—

Dr.: Go to hell?

Pt.: To go someplace. That's right. And yet I put myself out.

Dr.: I will see you next week.

*Exploration of her sense of discontent, irritability, and unhappiness
continues. It is established that she has an inner compulsion to be
good and has always been that way. Her need for order and perfec-*

tion began as a child and arose as a means of fending off her mother. In fact, fending off meant yielding and total acquiescence. The anger that mounts in such a situation provokes both guilt and fear of retaliation, thereby reinforcing the adaptive good behavior.

In this interview, the past origins of present behavior are clarified, and she is sympathetically supported in her struggles so that she can begin both to speak of and to become aware of inner feelings that she has always been afraid to know. We learn a good deal about her original family and the sources of present attitudes which are significant in the genesis and onset of her present dysfunction. The one person she does not fear is her husband, who clearly is felt to be, like her father, weak, nice, and totally dominated by mother. His compliance and helpfulness only increase her sense of guilt.

During the past week, the only medication she has been taking is that prescribed by the dermatologist for her urticaria. She was able to go out shopping with her two youngest children for the first time and also went alone to school on a matter about one of her children— another first. These gains were countered by marked anorexia and nausea. One may speculate (data is not available) whether the anorexia might be warding off angry, destructive oral fantasies which were aroused by the proposal that she takes no more pills, and whether the nausea might be an attempt to eject the bad mother introject (therapist) who places demands upon her. There is no question but that swift psychological movement has been set off. We see further refinement of the central issue in the rapid uncovering of typical conflicts of the obsessive-compulsive neurotic.

Third Interview

The interview begins with the patient complaining about her continuing insomnia, nausea, and anorexia. In addition, she describes a particularly severe anxiety attack over the previous weekend. I investigate the nausea and anorexia further, even to the point of inquiring whether she thought she might be pregnant. She is certain that she is not pregnant but does say that she feels as though she is having morning sickness constantly. Despite her complaints, she has the feeling that what she is experiencing is not due to physical causes but rather is a manifestation of her "nerves." She wonders if it might have something to do with her "trying to get used to being without the pills."

Dr.: . . . It's hard for you to go without the pills.
Pt.: It has been, but I managed. I managed to go out last weekend. I went to the hospital to see my mother a couple of times.
Dr.: Who did you go with?

Pt.: I took my daughter. I didn't go alone. But I came here alone on the bus.

Dr.: Really? The first time—

Pt.: Yeah—I made that much of a trip.

Dr.: How do you feel?

Pt.: I feel pretty good today.

Dr.: How did it feel being on the bus alone?

Pt.: Not too bad. We almost got hit by a car so that took up my time . . .

Dr.: The bus almost got hit?

Pt.: A car came toward the bus and he swerved. Everybody on the bus was talking, so I didn't mind it too much, and I was here before I knew it.

Dr.: Something that you are always afraid of almost happened.

Pt.: I know, but it didn't bother me. For days now I have been thinking of coming and getting on the bus because I knew I had to come alone. Like I said last week, worrying about things that are coming, and they haven't happened yet.

Dr.: Right.

Pt.: I managed to make it anyway.

Dr.: And nothing happened.

Pt.: That's right. So I will have to try again. The other thing this week was that strange feeling— . . . (*Despite her complaints, she is pleased to tell me of an important gain in coming alone to see me. The internal pressure felt by her to come alone in compliance with what she felt I wished for her to do is followed associatively with a renewed exploration by her of the severe anxiety attack she had suffered since her last visit with me. She reveals that she had rushed to the hospital to see her mother on the day of her last interview, rushed again on the next day to see her, and had the attack that night. She described what sounded like some forty-eight hours of almost frenzied rushing about—such frenzy that her husband yelled at her to take her time, that there was no need to rush.*) I don't have the time for everything. Hurry and have it done. I don't know why I did that Saturday. I had plenty of time.

Dr.: That may be, but you always do feel as though you are working against time.

Pt.: Time—yeah. Yesterday I happened to blow my top and I felt good ever since.

Dr.: What was that about? . . . (*There follows an incident in which her mother forced the patient to drop everything she was doing to come to the hospital immediately to pay a bill prior to mother's discharge from the hospital. The patient did as told but was able to tell her mother that she was through rushing about for her: "If you want things done hire yourself a secretary. I got that off my chest and felt better. I don't know where she thinks she is going that she has to have her bill marked paid."*) Where do you think she thinks she is going?

Pt.: I don't know, she—that's how she wants it done. Right away.

Dr.: You are the same way.

Pt.: I know. My daughter told me that yesterday. She said, "I don't know what you are complaining about because you are just like her." I said, "Oh, don't tell me that." "Well, you are. When you want something done it's got to be done just then."

Dr.: You don't like to hear that.

Pt.: No. I felt awful. I said, "The next time I do that"—and she said, "alright, next time you do it, I will tell you about it. I said, "Okay." That's the difference between her and me—we can talk like that or laugh about it after.

Dr.: That was your oldest?

Pt.: My oldest daughter. I figure if she has enough gumption in her, good luck to her. Nobody is going to walk all over her.

Dr.: You think she has the gumption that you didn't have.

Pt.: She'll get along better than I am getting along. She seems to manage.

Dr.: You don't think that you are getting along so well?

Pt.: Not as well as I would like to. Things could be changed. I probably could change my ways.

Dr.: You did tell your mother off yesterday.

Pt.: Well, not told her off in that sense. I tried to tell her in a nice way.

Dr.: How did she respond?

Pt.: She was tired and she didn't feel good, and I told her that I felt bad—I didn't feel good either but that she had already been taken care of and that I was still in the process of being taken care of. (*The identification with her mother emerges repeatedly: this time with special emphasis on the need to be taken care of.*)

Dr.: What did she say?

Pt.: That's true, but you don't know how I am going to turn out.

Dr.: What did she mean?

Pt.: She hasn't been feeling well. She is drawing her own conclusions as to what is wrong with her.

Dr.: What is that conclusion?

Pt.: She seems to think that she has cancer. Of course, we are not giving any information out. We feel that the less she knows the better for her, because she will dwell on it. So we tell her as much as we think she should know . . . (*Patient then tells that her mother is with her sister. Mother wanted to come to the patient's house, but sisters told her that patient had enough to do without having her there, too. She added that sisters told mother this in the presence of the doctor at the hospital, so that mother could not object too violently.*)

Dr.: So you were spared that—

Pt.: That burden. Of course, I am not spared the phone calls and the anxiety and the worrying. I have to chase down to my sister's place every chance I get.

Dr.: You go down to your sister's house to see your mother?

Pt.: I went down last night. I gave her a back rub and fixed her something to eat, and we sat and talked.

Dr.: You are so damned nice . . . Tell me, why did you go down there, run right down and pay, even though you know that bills can wait?

Pt.: I think I went more or less because I was so angry. My husband was furious with me. I told him I wouldn't do it again. He said, "You better, or I will tell her." I said, "No, I will tell her."

Dr.: Whose money did you use to pay the hospital?

Pt.: Money that my father had given me—that was set aside for her. Not my own. I don't have it.

Dr.: This is money your father left for—

Pt.: For her—in my name. So everything is in my name, and I have to do all the chasing . . .

Dr.: How come he left the money with you?

Pt.: I don't know. Like I say, I am the baby, but I have all the responsibility that you would think the older ones would have. But it doesn't really bother me that much. It's just a job. But don't push me—I will do it when I am ready.

Dr.: Yes, it may not be very important in itself. But as you told me, you are the youngest, but the greatest responsibility was placed on you.

Pt.: A burden or a responsibility.

Dr.: And I suppose it's because everybody somehow knew that . . .

Pt.: I suppose they figured that if I want to please her, go ahead.

Dr.: What do they all know about you?

Pt.: Oh, they knew that I was eager—I was an easy person, you know, to get to do everything. My sister told me, "Do you want to please her? Go ahead, but your life will be miserable."

Dr.: I guess they all knew that you were devoted to her.

Pt.: I was devoted, but they stood in their own fear at the same time.

Dr.: They all knew that you were devoted to her and that anything you were asked to do you would do, whether you would like it or not . . . (*But, although the patient is the devoted one to her, mother has let it be known that if anything happens to her all her possessions will go to her sons. Patient's sister defended the patient's right to inheritance because of her constant devotion. The patient denies that she would want anything of her mother's, primarily because its presence would be an additional reminder of mother's real presence. However, she is hurt by so evident a lack of reward. How does she feel about mother giving everything only to her brothers?*)

Pt.: She has a son complex, I call it. She is for her boys. Her girls can do everything for her, but her boys she idealizes. They very seldom come to see her.

Dr.: She thinks the boys—

Pt.: The sun rises and sets on them.

Dr.: Your mother has always looked on her sons in a different way than her daughters?

Pt.: Oh yeah, she was very partial to boys. Even in grandchildren, too.

Dr.: She doesn't think much of girls.

Pt.: Maybe she figures that we are there. She doesn't even have to think about it. She wants, and we are there.

Dr.: This is what you are for.

Pt.: It's the only thing that I can think of.

Dr.: You must like that.

Pt.: No, not actually. I hope that I never do it to my children. She will be collapsing and dying all over the place until this weekend when the boys come, and then she will be fine.

Dr.: You are telling me that your mother has never hesitated to use you.

Pt.: In a sense, that's it.

Dr.: But the rewards go to somebody else.

Pt.: I suppose she figures that is my obligation. I don't know. Obligation must stop somewhere.

Dr.: She certainly sounds like a very difficult woman. Now let's hear more about you ... (*She does not think that much has changed since the previous week. I remark on the fact that she had come by herself today and add that we should nevertheless consider further her lack of appetite and the nausea. We learn that she usually feels better at night and is able to eat a sandwich along with a few beers at that time. The nausea, she says, "is like morning sickness. Then it will stop at night. I have an easier time to eat at night than I do all day." She repeats her conviction that the nausea and lack of appetite has to do with her "nerves."*) I agree with you. So our job is to find out what there is about your nervousness that—

Pt.: I don't understand how I can wake up nervous. If I've slept any amount of time, I should be quieted down to some degree.

Dr.: As soon as you wake up, there it is.

Pt.: Every morning. I have the feeling that here is another day and then it just builds up and builds up.

Dr.: And then as the day draws on, you feel better?

Pt.: I feel better because I seemed to have gotten over that part of the day. It's over, and then it's alright, and I start feeling good.

Dr.: Well, this brings us back to think a little bit again about one of the things I mentioned to you the first time that we met. That you suffer this general sense of discontent, because now you are saying that when you get up in the morning, you think of the day ahead of you and it makes you feel sick. (*Back to the global central issue.*)

Pt.: I don't want to face the day.

Dr.: So you don't want to face the day.

Pt.: Each day is the same. It's the bickering with the little boy about playing, which he doesn't want to do, and he doesn't know what to do. He is bored, and there is nothing to do around the house. All of this is building up that he wants to go out on the street to play. (*Return to the central issue stimulates her to speak of a significant area of concern.*) He is four years old, and I don't want to let him go out, so he bickers with me all morning long. And I know that will go on, and I will have to face it until he is old enough to go to school. At 2:30 they are all going to start coming in and arguing about going out. I hate to hear them saying they are going out because I know the little boy is going to start up again. He wants to go. I let him go out yesterday and he almost got hit by a car.

Dr.: You are saying that when you think of each day, you are kind of sick and tired of your own boring existence. (*She has made it perfectly clear that she is so frightened about the boy getting hit by a car; my remark is to point up the evident contradiction that far from being bored, she is scared.*)

Pt.: I have the little one, and he is hard to handle. The others were never as active as he is, and you hate to let him go out the front door because you wouldn't want to see him under the wheels of a car. And that's how he is—he is so quick—so he is a constant worry until he goes to bed at night. And then you feel as if somebody is taking that log right off your shoulders, once you see him sleeping. He is a big worry.

Dr.: You are afraid that he is going to get killed?

Pt.: I am afraid that something is going to happen to him because he is so fearless. He goes out in the street and doesn't look either way. He just goes.

Dr.: Is there no place for him to play?

Pt.: We have a backyard, but he doesn't stay there for two minutes. He hops the fence and out front he goes. By the time I get out the door, he is gone and he is on the street.

Dr.: Does he run out in the road?

Pt.: He just goes right in the road and crosses the street, and as many times as I tell him no, and he promises—but then he sees a friend and he is gone. Yesterday my daughter said that he just missed a car. I made him come in, and I had to listen to him cry for two hours. So I guess that's what gets on my nerves—this crying and begging me to go— . . . (*Of course, there is real danger on the street for a little boy. However, one can hardly avoid the suspicion that the unconscious message of the mother to the boy is exactly opposite to her conscious concern, particularly since it is a matter of constant affective outbursts between them.*)

Dr.: Are you saying that when you get up in the morning you feel sick thinking about the day and that it is really about the little boy?

Pt.: I think it is because I know that I can't conquer him no matter what I say. He seems to pest me all the time. (*The need to "conquer," to have total control lest her own dangerous impulses get out of control.*)

Dr.: You have trouble controlling the boys?

Pt.: I don't know. I just figure that boys are more active than girls. Maybe I should have been more firm with them in the beginning.

Dr.: I suppose that you couldn't be as firm as you would have liked because boys are more important, you know.

Pt.: I guess that's why I let them get away with more. I would say boys are like that—and oh, well—

Dr.: Just like your mother would say. She always thought more highly of boys.

Pt.: She seemed to care more. She was more affectionate towards the boys.

Dr.: I wonder if you have some of this same attitude without realizing it.

Pt.: That I can't control the boys?

Dr.: Yes.

Pt.: I have been looking for ways to conquer them. I have tried everything, but I just don't get the best of them. They won't give in . . . If I could make the boys do what I like it would be fine. Not what I like, but obey and not give me too much to worry about.

Dr.: Tell me, did your brothers have their way with their mother? . . . (*I am weaving her past experience with the present in this regard since this is clearly an important, recurrent theme. Of course, her brothers were freer than she in all respects. She examines again the intensely felt inner compulsion to be nice and totally obedient to her mother. I remark that she acts like someone who has been conquered, so that even to this day the inner demand provokes great guilt if she tries to do something simply to suit herself. The present and past are brought to her attention once more as being the same when I remind her that she feels she has been conquered by her boys and how that gnaws at her.*)

Pt.: They do more than gnaw at me. They get me angry. When you have a four year old that you can't conquer, it's tough to face. And everybody can see it.

Dr.: Then you are a person who has been conquered. Would you agree to that? (*Repetition to make the point as well as to give the patient opportunity to defend herself further, or to come up with additional pertinent data.*)

Pt.: Yeah—by more than one, as you say.

THE CASE OF THE CONQUERED WOMAN

Dr.: And you don't like it. (*Help her identify her warded off feelings.*)
Pt.: No.
Dr.: It gets you.
Pt.: Yes, it gets me rather upset.
Dr.: We will look further next week.

In this third interview, she has already made some important gains in that she has been able to go out alone and even to come to her interview alone. She is pleased with herself for her progress, and this undoubtedly increases her self-esteem. Her very troublesome symptoms are explored—truly explored, because I move into them with her only so long as I feel that we are touching or reaching into useful data. If that seems not to be the case, I leave the path of inquiry and return to the central issue. Thus, we could make no progress in respect to the anxiety attack that she had during the preceding weekend. I felt that we must pursue the anorexia and nausea further since, in the absence of physical reasons (such as pregnancy), the unconscious dynamic in this phobic woman must be one of frightening oral sadistic fantasies and impulses toward fulfillment. The clue comes in the fact that as the day goes on she feels better, so that by night, she feels quite well again. We learn then that the symptoms serve to ward off her anxious fear in respect to her four-year-old son, with whom a reverberating relationship has been set up in connection with his wish to go out alone and her fear of what might happen to him. Unable to control him because she has unconscious wishes for him to be out of control, even as she would wish to be, she feels "conquered" by him. Thus, a central segment of her neurosis is revealed: the more she is able to control others, the more she feels in control of herself. Failing this, she is at the mercy of her own uncontrollable wishes, which she guards against by imposing phobic restrictions upon herself along with a series of somatic symptoms that turn her attention to herself. As she has been conquered by her mother, so she seeks to conquer her own children, especially the boys.

Her husband is "on a holiday" because she has let him know that she is going to be well in due course of time. This, like her gains, is a manifestation of the positive transference, with all its curative aspects. It is interesting to note that she says that she is the kind of person who is always working against time. This generalization can be made of all obsessionals and indicates the relevance of this method of treatment.

Fourth Interview

Dr.: (*Patient is sniffing.*) What's the matter?
Pt.: I have a nice cold. I don't know where I got it. The weather is so changeable. I have been pretty good this week.

Dr.: Pretty good means –

Pt.: Well, better than I have been. I've been going out. I haven't had many nervous thoughts. I've been eating, and I'm not nauseated any more.

Dr.: That's gone? (*Relief from nausea and anorexia follows discussion of her fears about letting her boy outside alone.*)

Pt.: Thank goodness. I seem to be more like myself—eating. But I am not sleeping. I'm still not sleeping.

Dr.: What do you mean not sleeping?

Pt.: I have a hard time falling asleep. But other than that I have been doing good.

Dr.: And what pills are you taking?

Pt.: None.

Dr.: Drinking much beer?

Pt.: No, not too much. Before I have my dinner or my supper, that's all.

Dr.: And you have been going out?

Pt.: Yes. I've been going out every night—going down to see my mother and to help my sister. And then I have been getting out with the children.

Dr.: Going out. When you go out at night who do you go with?

Pt.: Myself. It isn't too far—only a couple of blocks. I sit there for a couple of hours, and then I come home . . .

Dr.: And you are feeling better.

Pt.: I think that I am.

Dr.: What do you mean, you think. Don't you know?

Pt.: I think that I am a lot better than I think I was a week ago. I am not as nervous during the day, and I am able to get out with the children, which I haven't been able to do for awhile. And I am eating better . . .

Dr.: Do you remember anything that we talked about last week?

Pt.: I know we talked for a while about being aggravated with the children, I think.

Dr.: Since you were last here, did you find yourself thinking about anything that you or I had spoken about?

Pt.: Nothing other than the children bothering me. And I tried to overlook a lot of that.

Dr.: How were they bothering you?

Pt.: Oh, just around the house—just aggravating one another and fighting. So I didn't let it bother me. And I found myself putting them out whether it was cold or a little drizzle. They went out playing, whereas I used to make them stay in so that they wouldn't catch a cold . . . (*Note the passive compliance: "I found myself putting them out."*)

Dr.: Let me ask you this. During the course of the week, did you find yourself suddenly thinking anything that you and I talked about last week? (*Again directing the patient's attention to the central issue and to the associations that may appear in response to the transference.*)

Pt.: Well, like—during the course of the day, I think a lot about my visits.

Dr.: You do?

Pt.: Oh yes, I try to remember what is going on and try to correct it and overcome it. Gee, nothing specific.

Dr.: Anything at all, whether specific or not.

Pt.: I notice that my older son—I haven't let him bother me as much as he had been—different things that he would do. But he is punished, and he has to keep up with his punishment. I put my foot down a couple of times during the week.

Dr.: How do you punish him?

Pt.: He got a bad report card. He has to stay in and no television. He kept on asking me, "Can I go out, can I go out?" and I would say, "No," and that was it. I don't know what is happening with him or whether I am just being smart . . . (*She has been able to make a demand on her older son, even to inflict punishment, and is pleased with herself. For the first time she has not yielded to his arguments nor to his tears. We discuss her further thoughts and feelings about the boy. She feels that he does not take after her husband because "my husband isn't constructive, and my son likes to build things." She considers that the boy takes after her side of the family. He has a temper. As a matter of fact, all her children have a temper, and, unlike herself, they do not hold it back. She can be reasonable with them insofar as she does not look for perfection in the children. This is a statement of her conscious position. It is characteristic for the adult who has felt oppressed as a child to attempt consciously to avoid inflicting similar demands on her children. Unconsciously, the pressures are enormous both to repeat the same strictures and to encourage the kind of rebellion that was foreclosed to her as a child. The end result, of course, is to ensure the presence of the same conflict in the patient's present family as existed in her original one.*) I always said that I never could see a child that was perfect.

Dr.: You believed that you could be with your mother.

Pt.: No. I didn't really believe it, because I thought it was farfetched.

Dr.: But you tried to be what she wanted you to be.

Pt.: I remember when I was small, I would go through little tantrums if I couldn't go to anyplace that I wanted to.

Dr.: She said that you were perfect.

Pt.: She thought that I was a walking angel. She wouldn't hesitate to bring me anywhere. I hesitate to bring mine because they act up. They're not too bad, but it seems everyplace we go there are older people and they don't have the patience. (*In the presence of older people her own need to be bad must not be exposed by her children who must show that they, as she, are good.*)

Dr.: I take it that one of your chief aims has been that your kids will feel freer to speak up and not be like you, who were always keeping it inside yourself.

Pt.: I still find it hard to speak up. Things bother me, and I try to hold it back so as not to hurt somebody.

Dr.: You can see that?

Pt.: I can, and I feel that I am hurting somebody when I speak up.

Dr.: Really?

Pt.: I don't know why I should feel that way because my children don't hurt me when they speak up.

Dr.: That's right. So how do you account for that? You are afraid that if you speak up, you might hurt the other person—you have plenty of experience with your kids speaking up to you.

Pt.: It doesn't bother me because what they are speaking up about is a lot different than what I would be speaking up about.

Dr.: How would it be different?

Pt.: The subject would be different. What they speak up about is probably what they are wearing or what they want to do, and mine would be making me do something when I don't want to do it. I can't very well come back and say that I don't want to do it, but yet I have to do it.

Dr.: Like what?

Pt.: Different things. If I have to accommodate my sisters by helping out or do something that my mother wants.

Dr.: You wouldn't say no?

Pt.: No. I feel that I am learning to. My sister speaks up, but I can't.

Dr.: What would you say that would be hurtful?

Pt.: I feel that if my mother asks me to do something and I said no, I would feel like I was hurting her.

Dr.: She asks your sister and your sister says no. What happens to your mother. Is she hurt?

Pt.: She tells me about it—that my sister won't do this or that.

Dr.: Did she say that she was hurt?

Pt.: No, she wouldn't say she was hurt.

Dr.: So. Are you the one who hurts people if you say no?

Pt.: I don't know. I figure I am hurting, but I don't know.

Dr.: But you don't see the others—

Pt.: I know that she gets aggravated, probably angry, so I figure that she is hurt. So what they don't do, I do.

Dr.: It's very hard for you to say no. Do you think that you could say no to me?

Pt.: I don't know. I don't have an easy time saying no—as long as it isn't beyond my means—if it isn't something too tedious or strenuous.

Dr.: You mean that if it is something impossible, then you can say no.

Pt.: I would have to say no if it was impossible.

Dr.: But if it is something that you can do, you can't say no.

Pt.: If I can possibly do it, I'll say yes. But I know if I am asked to do something, and I have to take care of the children or something—well, then I turn around and say that I can't do it at that time, and when I have a free— a free time, then I will do it. Sometimes that goes over alright.

Dr.: I gather from what you have been saying that you are the kind of person that even with people who aren't so close to you, like your mother or your sisters, maybe even in your social group, you would find it hard to say no.

Pt.: Like in a group or anything, and they ask would I do this? Would I bake this? Would I do that?

Dr.: You say yes.

Pt.: I would say yes. I might gripe about it all the time I am doing it.

Dr.: I am sure.

Pt.: And probably hate doing it, but I will do it.

Dr.: And you say yes because you are afraid that you will hurt the person.

Pt.: Yes. That's the feeling I have.

Dr.: Mrs. Smith asks you to bake a cake for this particular party, and you don't really want to, but you will say yes because you don't want to—

Pt.: Hurt her.

Dr.: Hurt her feelings. But how do you feel when you say yes?

Pt.: It depends. If I am not too wrapped up with something that I have to do at home, I don't mind doing it. But if I'm busy—

Dr.: But when you say yes at a time when you really want to say no?

Pt.: No?

Dr.: How do you feel?

Pt.: Well, I feel kind of confused. I wish that I didn't have to. I don't know whether I am coming or going. I would be betwixt and between. I will have to put my mind to that and push something aside at home to accomplish that one thing.

Dr.: So how do you feel about that?

Pt.: Then I know that I start building up when I start—whatever I am pushing aside I will have double to do later—so then I get all nervous. But when it's all done it's over with.

Dr.: But you do get nervous.

Pt.: I say never again. But I find that the next time, I do it again.

Dr.: And you do get all tense, irritable.

Pt.: Last week my daughter came in and says will you bake a cake for school? I said no, and I didn't bake it. That was the first time since they have been going to school that I have said no.

Dr.: What happened?

Pt.: When I said no, it was no. So she didn't bother me. It didn't bother me saying no that time because I had too much to do.

Dr.: But if you are asked to do something—we will use the example of Mrs. Smith—bake a cake for the group, and you say yes because you can't say no when you really don't want to do it, you go home and you do it. Don't you get tense and nervous—irritable about it?

Pt.: I bake the cake, and yet I would just like to throw it at anything. No matter how good it will come out, I don't feel that I have accomplished anything . . . (*Obviously, I am pushing and prodding her to come to terms with the kind of feeling that she has when demands are made of her. She acknowledges her wish to throw the cake but then automatically pays for her bad feeling by devaluing her baking. The constant inner demand is that she sacrifice her own wishes in favor of doing for others. Her husband recognizes this and berates her for giving up a ceramics class that she had been taking and, as one might guess, immediately relates the sacrifice to the felt demands of the mother that the patient spend more evenings with her. She fears that mother might think that the patient thought less of mother if she not only did not meet all of mother's demands, but also was devoting some evenings to her own pleasure. She consoles herself with the statement that she is "conquering" one thing for herself by going out alone, even if it is to mother's home.*) Myself—I think that I have gotten to the point where I am disgusted with all the chasing, being ordered, being asked to do this, being asked to do that.

Dr.: For you, to be asked is like an order.

Pt.: Because I don't want to do it. I could stay home and wash walls and it wouldn't bother me as much because I would be doing something that I want to do.

Dr.: You decided that you—

Pt.: Want to do. Yesterday I was tired, so I didn't feel good when I got down there. I told her I wouldn't be in so much. She didn't say anything, but I know what she was thinking.

Dr.: Of course, if you are sick, that gives you a good excuse.

Pt.: I tell her that I am tired. Then she knows that I have gone out or something. She will say, "Why did you go out if you were sick?" I just say I am tired—I leave it at that.

Dr.: Has your husband ever said anything much about this business between you and your mother?

Pt.: No. He is getting more or less aggravated with the idea of me going out every night. He thinks I should have more time to myself.

Dr.: When did he begin to think this way?

Pt.: This week, when I went out every night except Tuesday. He thought that was too much. She goes for her checkup, and if she's alright, I'll stop going down.

Dr.: Has he ever spoken before about this business of people asking you to do all the time?

Pt.: Yeah. He will always say, "Why can't you say no?" I never have an answer.

Dr.: Well, you have one answer. You are always afraid that if you say no, the other person will get hurt.

Pt.: The feeling that I have hurt somebody. I don't like to hurt anybody. Some people don't care what they say or do—as long as they do what they want, they don't care who is affected by it. But I can't be like that. (*Although her fear that if she says no someone will be hurt clearly points up the extent of her unconscious rage, she is much too defended to allow for any kind of adequate exploration of this side of her feelings. In turn, the vigor of her defense dictates caution in the face of feelings that are intensely intolerable to her. I turn, therefore, to another more acceptable mode of examining her concern in respect to her own hostility.*)

Dr.: Isn't there another way of looking at that. It's true, you know, that to hurt people for the hell of it is not a very nice thing, but if you are the kind of person who thinks that if you say no this will hurt the other person, might it not be that you are the kind of person who is afraid that she won't be liked?

Pt.: It could be.

Dr.: Do you think that you are the kind of person who has a special need to be liked?

Pt.: Maybe. I like to be wanted. I like to be accepted in groups or whoever is around. I wouldn't want to be shunned . . . (*The fear of being "shunned," rejected, confirms so much her own feeling of badness as to make compliance an imperative. She speaks of a descending order of comfort in dealing with others; most comfortable with those she does not "have to do much for," less comfortable with her children and least comfortable with her mother. However, since there is little to choose from between her feelings about her mother and about her own family, she readily moves on to repeat the issue of whether she is beginning to conquer her older son or whether he remains in charge.*) Oh, he has conquered me a long time ago. But now I am turning the other way. I am starting to conquer him, I hope. In the one weekend, I have seen a difference.

Dr.: One of the things that has upset you and made you feel discontented is that you have felt conquered. How does somebody feel who can't say no?

Pt.: Like I always say to my husband, I don't know where you get these definitions. It feels like you are drowning and you can't save yourself. I don't know how to put it.

Dr.: Is that the way you put it to your husband?

Pt.: Yeah. As an example. There is no hope. There is no way out that—

Dr.: It means that you are helpless, like a drowning person.

Pt.: That's the only way I can put it when I know that I can't get the best of him.

Dr.: Or the best of your mother, for example.

Pt.: Well, I notice that I speak up more than I did.

Dr.: But you have often felt like a drowning person.

Pt.: Even in an argument. No matter what it was about, I never could win. She would always get the last word. Then I take it out on my husband and children.

Dr.: You have a way of expressing yourself very clearly.

Pt.: Well, this is like the comparisons. You have to make them sound so morbid sometimes. Well, that's how I feel, and my husband can't understand it.

Dr.: When you bake a cake because you are asked to do it even if you don't want to, you do it but you would like to take that cake and throw it.

Pt.: My husband says when you get that mad just throw it. That's childish.

Dr.: And you remember that you once said that if your mother came in the house and saw that it was dirty—

Pt.: Upset.

Dr.: You said that would kill her. Now we hear that sometimes you get to feel like a drowning person. Demands are made on you and you can't say no. So you do have very strong feelings and emotions, don't you? Can't tell by looking at you.

Pt.: Well, I feel it. I would like to say no. I often wonder how things would be if I said no as many times as I felt like it.

Dr.: You would have a picnic for a while, wouldn't you?

Pt.: I would either have a picnic for a while, or I would have everybody hating me—one of the two.

Dr.: That is one of your concerns, isn't it? . . . Have you thought of yourself as having very strong emotions?

Pt.: Like getting upset?

Dr.: I mean, really feel—

Pt.: If I got real angry, nine times out of ten I will sit down and probably cry about it, and I will get it out of my system that way.

Dr.: Did you ever feel like killing somebody?

Pt.: No.

Dr.: Never?

Pt.: No. Actually killing, or saying it? Because I say that all day long. I will say, "I will kill you," and you shouldn't say that because the children don't know what you mean. I wouldn't wish anybody ill or anything. I couldn't— I could dislike a person and not wish them any harm.

Dr.: Have you ever hated anybody?

Pt.: No, not in that sense of the word. Disliked, aggravated, but I never hated anyone.

Dr.: No matter what has gone wrong or what has happened you have never—

Pt.: No, I don't think I have really been hurt enough to hate anybody. Nobody has really hurt me that much.

Dr.: You never hated anybody even for a moment? In a moment of anger?

Pt.: Maybe in a moment of anger. I could never keep a grudge and hate a person. I don't like family friction where they don't speak to one another. That bothers me. Like, my sister doesn't talk to my brother. I am always trying to push them together . . . (*Her feeling of drowning allows me to amplify in terms of her feelings of helplessness. Thus, we have been able to move more closely to her deeply painful negative feelings, and I have been given a green light to pursue these more closely. She sees herself very much in the role of peacemaker in both families.*)

Dr.: It's all very nice, and it's nice to have people around who don't hate, or bear grudges—that's really very nice.

Pt.: That's how I try to teach my children, but they have different feelings. They get aggravated with one another, and they say harsh words. They hate one another—"I hope you get hit by a car"—then I go to pieces. I like to see everybody get along.

Dr.: So you are the kind of person who usually feels in such situations that there is nothing much that you can do but agree or give in—or feel, as you said, like a drowning person. A person must feel pretty damned desperate—

Pt.: You aren't kidding. It can get aggravating.

Dr.: More than aggravating—desperate.

Pt.: And then you look for help, and sometimes you can't get the help.

Dr.: What do you do?

Pt.: I get over it, but it takes a long time.

Dr.: You get nervous, tense, and scared—irritable.

Pt.: Very irritable. Everything bothers me. At times it feels hopeless when it has happened—whatever went on.

Dr.: How does a hopeless person feel?

Pt.: As if there isn't anything to look for the next day, you know there is nothing there, until you see that there is something there.

Dr.: Ever feel like dying?

Pt.: When I feel sick I always say that I think I am going to die, but I don't want to die.

Dr.: But it does build up inside of you.

Pt.: It builds up and I—

Dr.: Get this desperate, hopeless feeling, and you don't know what to do about it. Might say that at a time like that you really feel entirely conquered.

Pt.: That's when I feel I wish I were away from everybody. Just my husband and my children.

Dr.: Just with your husband and your children and leaving—

Pt.: Leave my family.

Dr.: Which family?

Pt.: My family. My mother. Just get away from everybody that is arguing or bickering.

Dr.: It is hard to get away from your mother, isn't it?

Pt.: No matter where you go your conscience is with you, so if she isn't there you figure—

Dr.: She is always with you.

Pt.: If she isn't there physically, I feel the stress and the strain just the same.

Further elaboration about her feeling of being conquered and how she cannot say no out of fear that she will hurt the other person. She knows that people can say no to her without her suffering severe pain, but this does not alter her fear of hurting others. When asked if she could say no to me, she was hesitant, said that she didn't think she could say no to me but I detected a very subtle glance that said, "if you want me to say no, I'll say it." She can say no if she has reality to support her. She will always give up of her own time to do for others. It is in this setting that she becomes increasingly tense, anxious, and irritable. This can lead to the feeling of being so overwhelmed as to feel "like a drowning person," helpless and desperate.

Symptomatically, she has improved further. Her appetite is normal again and she goes in and out of her home alone. Some insomnia is still present, but she feels less tense and less put upon, with some beginning feeling that she may master the people in her environment.

In this fourth interview, the transference, concealed very much in her need to be compliant, continues to exercise its positive influence.

Fifth Interview

The patient had to wait at the pay desk of the clinic and is immediately concerned about whether or not she is late for her appointment with me. She has a cold and is impelled to tell me that she has taken aspirin for it but continues to remain off any other medications. Her children are ill, but she has nevertheless gone out alone several nights. She came alone to her appointment today and is pleased with her feeling that "maybe I am conquering that." She will test herself further by not returning directly to her home, but giving herself the pleasure of going shopping.

Dr.: ... You are making progress.

Pt.: I think that I am. I mean, I feel that I can change something, which I haven't felt in a long time. I have the children around, but I haven't had the feeling that I needed them for security or anything. It's not the thing to need security from children. I have managed pretty good, I think. I don't know what anybody else thinks, but if I feel like I feel, that's the important part.

Dr.: Do you concern yourself as to what others think about you?

Pt.: Not right now, I don't.

Dr.: What do you mean not right now?

Pt.: I used to.

Dr.: Did you?

Pt.: Yeah. I mean, my husband used to say you are doing good and I didn't believe him, but I feel different now.

Dr.: Now if he says you are doing good, you believe him.

Pt.: I know I am. Maybe I'm too confident now—one extreme to another—but I feel that way. Nervous at times, but not bad. I seem to be accepting it more or less.

Dr.: So you have a good feeling . . . When was the last time you can recall feeling so good?

Pt.: As good as I felt this week? I would say maybe a few years. I never had the urge that I wanted to go out, or I wanted to do anything, but now I feel I want to do things.

Dr.: And you're planning to do that?

Pt.: I hope so.

Dr.: Like going shopping after you leave here today . . . How long are you going to be out?

Pt.: I will be home to fix dinner. That will be enough for one day. Last week we were talking about my saying no. I kept thinking of that all weekend. I have to remember because every week I come, you ask what we talked about. I had the opportunity to say no. It turned out that there were two wakes that I didn't want to go to, and I didn't go.

Dr.: Two wakes.

Pt.: Yes, which I don't care to go to anyways. The immediate family has to go, so I just didn't go. That's as good as saying no. Other times I used to drag myself and go, and I would be depressed when I got home. I just told my husband, "I am not going." He didn't question me, and he went by himself. So that's one thing I did.

Dr.: So you did your homework.

Pt.: I did a little homework. It seems like a lot to me. I don't know if it is or not, but it was an effort.

Dr.: Is it of some concern to you that I asked you to think about what we had been talking about, and that you have to remember?

Pt.: I was concerned that I didn't remember exactly the conversation.

Dr.: What was your worry about?

Pt.: That I couldn't remember. I didn't know whether I was just lax in trying to remember, or was I blocking it out. I just didn't know why I wasn't remembering, because I can remember other things that are going on.

Dr.: Do you think that if you don't remember that you might displease me?

Pt.: I didn't know whether I was supposed to be able to remember, so all week I kept saying, "I have to remember, I have to remember."

Dr.: All week you thought to yourself, "You have to remember, you have to remember."

Pt.: I kept saying that something would come up that would aggravate me, and I should say no—or should I say yes—but the occasion didn't arise.

Dr.: But when you thought to yourself that you have to remember, you have to remember, were you also thinking that after all, that you have to remember because Dr. Mann is going to be asking you?

Pt.: Asking me—like a job. If I were working I would have to remember different things that I would have to do.

Dr.: If you were working, that's true. But whose benefit are we here for?

Pt.: Mine.

Dr.: Yeah, so whose job is it?

Pt.: Mine.

Dr.: And—

Pt.: Yours. But I am the one who has to remember.

Dr.: You have to? For whose purposes?

Pt.: For my own.

Dr.: For your own, or for me?

Pt.: Well both. You are asking me, so I should remember.

Dr.: Suppose I ask you and you don't remember.

Pt.: I just have to say I don't remember. But I figure it displeases you that I am not progressing if I don't remember.

Dr.: Do you make progress to please me or to please you?

Pt.: I have to please you. I figure I am helping myself and I am putting my mind to it rather than leaving here and blanking my mind out.

Dr.: You feel that you have to please me.

Pt.: Not please you but probably what would be best for myself. Like being sick. You have to do things yourself whether you like it or not, and it helps. I realize that part.

Dr.: Are you saying, then, that sometimes you kind of hear my voice saying, "you have to remember, you have to remember?"

Pt.: No.

Dr.: It's your voice.

Pt.: It's my own. But I am supposed to, I should.

Dr.: You should.

Pt.: For my own good. I should think of myself, and this is part of my sickness, and I have to try and conquer it.

Dr.: For your own—

Pt.: My own good. Medication, in one sense of the word.

Dr.: But at the same time, you don't want to take any chances of displeasing me.

Pt.: I guess I don't like to displease anybody. That's my way, and I don't know if I change. I just don't like to hurt people.

Dr.: You mean that if you don't do as you think I want you to do that I will be hurt.

Pt.: I feel you are giving up time to try and help me. At least I could try and help myself.

Dr.: Well, that is certainly a very helpful way for you to look at it. But who are you going to do it for. For you? Or in order not to hurt me?

Pt.: No, for myself.

Dr.: You're sure now.

Pt.: Mmmm. Because I feel that's what you want me to do—for myself.

Dr.: Not for me.

Pt.: I figure that if I am displeasing you it's still connected with me because I am not doing what I should do for myself. You are not being hurt by it, but I am probably hurting myself.

Dr.: Except that you would be afraid that you might be hurting me.

Pt.: Not really. Wasting your time. You try to help me, and I should try to help myself—which I have been trying to do.

Dr.: That's certainly true. But it's very difficult for you to displease. What's going to happen if you find yourself in a position here where you will have to say no to me for one reason or another?

Pt.: Maybe as time goes on, I am hoping to get that courage and the demand to say to somebody eventually—

Dr.: It takes courage.

Pt.: Everything that I have been asked of I have been able to fulfill. There will be a day when I probably won't be able to, and I will have to say no. I hope I have the courage to say no when the time comes.

Dr.: You say that it takes courage to say no. That means that you are afraid.

Pt.: I am not always afraid to say no. Like I mentioned last week, if I feel that I can't do something, then I can say no. If I don't say no, it's because I feel I can do it, so why not do it. But then I have a voice behind me saying, "You don't want to do it, what are you doing it for?" I just don't want to say no. It isn't a fear. I can't explain it. If I make somebody happy, then I am happy myself.

Dr.: Where did you learn this from—this whole idea of trying to make everybody happy?

Pt.: I don't know. It wasn't at home.

Dr.: It wasn't at home.

Pt.: No. I never saw anybody put themselves out of their way to make anything extra happy. What everybody did they had to do, and that was it.

Dr.: I think it's a very good way to be—to help people and make people happy as long as it doesn't have it's effect on you. You didn't learn it at home.

Pt.: No, I don't think that I did.

Dr.: Your mother hasn't been that way.

Pt.: My mother did what she had to do, like most parents. Certainly not to please me.

Dr.: Your father?

Pt.: I don't remember. Not putting himself out for us. He used to put himself out for friends, I know. He seemed more happy outside than he did at home. I don't know why, but I remember that much . . . (*The long foregoing excerpt, simple in its style, is extremely important. She displays very vividly her current adaptive mode, the imperative demands of her never-relenting superego and the transference exposure of the genesis of her fear of hurting by saying no. My interventions aim at pressing the patient to confront herself with the inappropriateness of her inner demands as she experiences them with me. Of course, she did not learn to be compliant by identifying in this respect with her mother. In other words, she is not so excessively nice because her mother served as a model. Her father, while not demanding of her and, in fact, very much an object of oppression by mother, too, managed his relationship with mother by withdrawal. She then does tell something of how she came to adopt her particular adaptive and defensive style. She tells that mother made father miserable and why.*) I think she just wanted a perfect husband, and you don't always get a perfect person. She always thought she was perfect and everybody else should be.

Dr.: Well she made you perfect.

Pt.: In her eyes. Not mine.

Dr.: You tried.

Pt.: Mmmm, I tried, but I knew I was doing it because she wanted me to, not because I wanted to, so I felt guilty there . . . (*We see now that her adaptive style has arisen out of a defensive identification with the aggressor. Unable to cope with her conflicting responses to mother's demands, she finds a solution by becoming like her mother in respect to the most painful and most aggressive aspect of the mother's personality, that is, to demand perfection.*)

Dr.: Would you ever go out of the house the way your father did, you know, in order to get away?

Pt.: Most of the time.

Dr.: When did you?

Pt.: I would go out with my girl friends—go to a dance or to the movies. Then when I had boy friends I—which always proved difficult because they never met with her approval.

Dr.: None of them?

Pt.: No. Nobody was perfect enough for her daughters. She just brought up perfect daughters. But we all managed to get out anyway, and now she needs her son-in-laws even though she once frowned on them.

Dr.: Your father had to get out in order to enjoy himself more; you did, too, and again your sisters.

Pt.: More or less.

Dr.: How about your brothers?

Pt.: Oh, no. My brothers didn't have a hard time. Whatever they did was alright. They didn't have to go out; they brought the girls home. If we brought the boys home, they weren't accepted.

Dr.: They weren't welcome.

Pt.: No, but they managed to come. They were stubborn if they wanted us, so they kept coming and taking the arguments that were with it.

Dr.: Arguments?

Pt.: She discussed everything they said. Something she didn't like, she would get into an argument. They didn't give up. I wouldn't put up with it if I didn't have to.

Dr.: You put up with a lot, didn't you?

Pt.: I think that I did more than I feel that I should have. I feel that I have done as much as I could be expected to do. I told my husband that I am not doing anymore because there is a limit to what you can do. I stopped and looked around, and I feel that I am pushing aside my own family for my mother, which I shouldn't do . . . (*Note the transition from the past to the present—the recurrent central issue. There follows a discussion of her mother's illness. The diagnosis of a malignant tumor has been made, and the patient expects her to live another three to six months. "She is probably dying, but if you give in to her you will be nothing but a mop until she is gone, which isn't going to leave a loving memory." Thus, she shows intuitive awareness of the fact that mother's death will expose her to the hateful side of her feelings about her. Note, too, how regularly the patient speaks of herself by saying "you" rather than "I." This may be understood as a means of distancing herself from the acceptance of responsibility for what she is saying. It is of equal importance to understand it as an expression of the constant presence of the internalized voice of her mother saying, "you do this, you do that." She has been thinking a good deal about her mother's illness and confesses to the thought that she had wished mother would die in the operation rather than live and suffer. "I don't want to seem ungrateful for anything that she had done for me—it's not that I am wishing her dead." The question has arisen whether mother will ask to live with the patient after leaving the hospital. The patient is determined that this shall not happen.)* Well, they are not going to bring her to me if it's going to get worse, because I can't take it with the children. My sister can't please. Nobody can please.

Dr.: But are you prepared to say no?

Pt.: I have already said no.

Dr.: But she might turn on the heat.

Pt.: No—no—impossible. It wouldn't be fair to the children. I mean, they know her the way she was, and she wasn't that happy a grandmother that you would like to remember her anyway. I wouldn't want them to see her miserable and suffering because I imagine she is going to get a lot worse than she ever was. As miserable as I am, I could never be like she is with the children.

Dr.: Does your sister understand that your mother is dying?

Pt.: Yes, but she is kind of burying her head in the sand. She is always hoping for a miracle to come around the corner.

Dr.: And your brothers—they know all about this?

Pt.: They only call her on the telephone, and there is only so much you can tell because she is always around. My sister doesn't want them to know too much. She doesn't want them coming down. Then she would get suspicious.

Dr.: If they visit her?

Pt.: If they visit her too much. One of them doesn't come at all.

Dr.: So if he comes, then she knows that this is her last—

Pt.: That her time is up—if he shows up . . .

Dr.: I gather from what you have been saying that it sounds as though you are— how shall I put it—becoming a free citizen again.

Pt.: Well, I feel that half the load is off my shoulders.

Dr.: Half?

Pt.: I feel I am coming along.

Dr.: What is the other half?

Pt.: Well, in due time I figure that will fall off, too, I hope.

Dr.: What do you mean by the other half? Half is off. What is the other half?

Pt.: Well, when I don't have to come anymore then I will feel that I have conquered myself instead of everybody else conquering—

Dr.: When you don't have to come where?

Pt.: When I don't have to come for help anymore.

Dr.: Here. So half the load is right here.

Pt.: I said to my husband—it's an awful thing to say—"I am getting help, and I go. And I wish I could just take the other bus and go shopping instead. Yet I wouldn't want to say anything to hurt Dr. Mann, but that's how I feel." I don't know if that's right. I feel that I wish I didn't have to come.

Dr.: Of course, you don't know if that's right. It is your feeling.

Pt.: I mean that I know I am getting help, and I appreciate it—the help I am getting—but deep down I wish I could go somplace else. I feel—shopping would make me happy.

Dr.: You mean there are things that you could be doing that you would enjoy more than coming here.

Pt.: That's right. Like my husband says, "Gee, you shouldn't take that attitude. You are getting help." I said, "I know that I'm getting help, but"—

Dr.: It's like going to the dentist.

Pt.: You are going to get another toothache, but you don't want to go.

Dr.: You were afraid to tell me that.

Pt.: It bothered me to say that.

Dr.: Fear that it would hurt me?

Pt.: I said this morning before I left, "I am going to mention it," because it was on my mind, and I felt I would get it off my mind.

Dr.: You could think of better things you could do with your time.

Pt.: Than be coming here.

Dr.: Of course.

Pt.: Of course, if I didn't need the help I wouldn't be coming.

Dr.: That's half the load that you were saying that you have to manage yet. Do you think that you will have trouble with me?

Pt.: I don't think so. I found it easier coming than I thought I would. I thought I would find it difficult speaking. Like my husband said, "Do you mind the cameras and everything?" I said, "It doesn't bother me as long as I am going to get help." He thought I would be a different person and not want anyone to know, but I don't care.

Dr.: What did you tell him about the cameras?

Pt.: I don't even think about them. He asked me where they are. He makes a big joke out of it—television star. I have had a couple of people remark, "Don't you mind everybody knowing?" I said, "I haven't committed murder. I don't have anything to hide." (*Unconscious guilt-laden fantasies are expressed in seeming innocent denials.*)

Dr.: You have told others?

Pt.: I told one girl. She is going for help herself. I told her it's very nice out here. I don't know why she won't go here, but she has to go to her own doctor. I said, "It's up to you," but I am not like that.

Dr.: Did you tell her that you are on TV, too?

Pt.: No. I just told her that I think—I don't know what it is—recordings or—

Dr.: The doctors are watching over television.

Pt.: I said that it was on film. She thought that was terrible. I suppose it depends on what you have to talk about.

Dr.: What would be terrible about that?

Pt.: I imagine if somebody tried to hide that they murdered somebody that they wouldn't want to be talking about it.

Dr.: You haven't murdered anybody, have you?

Pt.: No!

Dr.: You might have wanted to, but you never did it.

Pt.: Well, I imagine that someone who has a guilt complex that they were trying to hide something—I have nothing to hide. I would just like to bare it all and get rid of it.

Dr.: You mean that you are not concerned as to who hears what you have to say?

Pt.: I am not of the old claim that you had to put all of this away and just lock the door—that it was a terrible thing to have somebody who was disturbed or mentally sick.

Dr.: Of course, when you first started here with me and I mentioned the TV cameras, I asked you if you minded, and you said no. But I don't think you could have said that you did mind it.

Pt.: I knew beforehand, and I wouldn't have come if I did mind it.

Dr.: You saw Dr. R., and she told you that—offered that I would see you and we would be on TV. Could you have said no to her at that point—"I don't want cameras and all that sort of thing?"

Pt.: No. If I said no I think I probably wouldn't need the help to begin with.

Dr.: Good point.

Pt.: I would be overconfident at that point.

Dr.: You had to say yes to her.

Pt.: I said yes because I didn't care who listened or watched. I wanted help. Like I say, I have my problems, but I don't think they are out of the ordinary, and they are not that deep and secretive.

Dr.: In other words, you think you are quite human.

Pt.: I imagine that other people have had domineering mothers and fathers.

Dr.: Oh, yes. But some domineering mothers and fathers are more domineering than others.

Pt.: That's true.

Dr.: You have had a rough one.

Pt.: I don't need anybody to tell me. I felt it. I mean, I could see it, and each crisis I could feel it coming on. It was always a crisis. If there was a baby coming, that was always a battle. There was never anything happy, like with some parents. All I had to say was that I was pregnant, and they were all up in arms . . . (*She tells now that with each pregnancy after the first, her sisters and mother would groan and object because of the patient's need for support through her pregnancy. She is too Catholic to allow for any contraceptive method other than rhythm. How harsh are the demands of her superego may be seen in the fact that she does not believe that her mother would at this point in history hesitate for a moment to use a contraceptive. Her husband has no overwhelming objections to such devices; it is only she who does.*)

Dr.: I want to remind you that you did mention something that was very important—that to a certain extent, half the load is gone. You are half free, and there is another half.

Pt.: If I could drop that—I feel good now.

Dr.: You mean that when you drop the other half then you will feel still better?

Pt.: One hundred percent.

The patient looks very well and is feeling very well, the best in at least ten years. She is off all medication, came alone for her interview, and is to go shopping alone directly after it. These are all impressive gains. In the usual short forms of psychotherapy, serious consideration would be given at this point to concluding the treatment. The patient is very much better and even says herself that if she didn't have to come anymore, she would then feel "one hundred percent." However, so much of the theme of the interview displays her inordinate need to acquiesce to the therapist in terms almost precisely applicable to her mother that the conclusion that the patient is ready to flee treatment, given the signal, is apparent. Even then, she needs to be given the signal; she cannot do it on her own. Therapy has become a burden almost as much as mother is a burden. Thus, there is ample evidence for the presence of a concealed negative transference in which she has "acquiesced" to becoming better and, having done so, wishes to be relieved of the therapy and therapist as burdens like her mother. In acquiescing to become better—that is, free of symptoms and off drugs—unconscious fantasies about the power of the early mother lend impetus both to the wish to acquiesce and to the expectation of omnipotent performance and fulfillment. In this fifth interview, she reveals a remarkable awareness of her ambivalence in respect to me. Half the load is off her shoulders, and I am the other half that burdens her. However, she does not wish to hurt me by telling me that she wished she did not have to come to see me. Note, too, the thin border in her mind, and particularly in her feelings, between hurting someone and murdering someone. Her reluctance to say no becomes very much more understandable when viewed in light of the deep-seated rage that makes any negative affect murderous.

Sixth Interview

Pt.: I have had a bad week.

Dr.: Really?

Pt.: Yeah. And I didn't feel too good coming over. I wasn't going to come.

Dr.: You weren't going to come at all?

Pt.: No, I felt so bad I took a cab.

Dr.: What's the matter?

Pt.: I don't know—just jumpy. I haven't been sleeping, and I am getting depressed over that. I didn't sleep at all last night.

Dr.: Been feeling jumpy all week—and unable to sleep?

Pt.: I can't sleep. I sleep maybe an hour or two, but I am up at three and four in the morning.

Dr.: Tell me all about it . . . (*Beginning five days prior to her present visit, she awakened feeling hot, perspiring, and having a sense of difficulty in breathing. Accompanying these was a generalized shakiness. When pressed further, she described a pain in the back of her head, "like a pressure," as being another part of the syndrome. She suddenly added that she was having the sense of pressure in her head as she sat with me: "I have it now— it's like a pressure—it feels hot, and I feel like I am going to pass out." The fear that she would pass out was so great that she had come by cab to see me rather than by bus, as usual.*) And you have that feeling now in your head?

Pt.: I have this pressure in the back of my head.

Dr.: And does your head feel hot?

Pt.: Mmmmm. It's an odd feeling like in the back of my neck . . .

Dr.: Are you scared?

Pt.: Scared? Well, I don't know what is going to happen. I wouldn't say really frightened because I don't know if it is going to go away or going to stay.

Dr.: And if it stays that way?

Pt.: It's uncomfortable.

Dr.: I am sure of that. But in addition to being uncomfortable, you are afraid something will happen.

Pt.: Mmmmm. I can't concentrate on anything. I just seem to be thinking of that, and that seems to take over all my thoughts.

Dr.: This that you feel in your head.

Pt.: It isn't something that you push out of your mind and try to—

Dr.: Tell me more of what it's like in your head.

Pt.: It's a hot feeling—it's not a sharp pain—it's like pressure—like somebody is pushing on it.

Dr.: As though someone is—

Pt.: Pushing.

Dr.: Pushing?

Pt.: On the back of my head. When it goes away, it feels like everything is just— the heat is—the heat is just coming down.

Dr.: Maybe that's important. The feeling is as though—as though somebody is pushing on the back of your head.

Pt.: And then sometimes it gets so bad I feel like my head is going to burst open. But that's when I first came in the clinic—that's what I came for. This is the second time that it's happened since then.

Dr.: Tell me more about this pushing on the back of your head. It feels like someone is pushing—

Pt.: It feels like my head would come forward if I didn't hold it back. My head feels heavy.

Dr.: *Now* what do you think about that?

Pt.: I don't know what to think about it. I was worried when I first had it. When the doctor examined me, it sort of put my mind at ease. I tried to keep saying, "It's all right; it will pass." But there was always that little doubt that maybe there is something wrong, and you keep thinking that . . .

Dr.: Did you have this strange feeling last night?

Pt.: I did. I had it around—this morning, around five.

Dr.: Where was it?

Pt.: I was sitting in the bedroom with the little boy.

Dr.: And what happened?

Pt.: I started to get this hot feeling and the pressure in the back of my head. I felt nauseated and dizzy. Then I woke up my husband. And then my arms get like pins and needles, numb.

Dr.: When was the last time that you had this thing with your head?

Pt.: Last month.

Dr.: Before I began to see you, or after?

Pt.: I think it was the first week, the first visit. It's just around a month be- cause my husband was remarking that it seems once a month I get like this. He said, "Maybe it has something to do with your period." But like he says, I just can't seem to let it go at that, and I dwell on it. I probably make more out of it than I should.

Dr.: Are you having your period?

Pt.: No. It's next week.

Dr.: Before your period, and your period is due next week.

Pt.: That's how I was the last time, too, just about a week before.

Dr.: And how long did it last the last time?

Pt.: Until I had my period, and then it left.

Dr.: If it comes on a week before your period, then it means there is a certain tension that you have. That's where you are now. But I don't suppose that helps you very much, does it?

Pt.: Not much because it seems like an eternity—just a week.

Dr.: And it's frightening.

Pt.: Like I said to my husband, "How long can you go without sleeping?" He said, "You shouldn't think that way." But when you are tired you can get awfully funny ideas—you would just like to sleep forever. So then he got disturbed because I was talking like that.

Dr.: He got disturbed because you were saying—

Pt.: Because I was getting discouraged, and I said I would rather be dead than be in this position. (*The patient describes now what seems very much to be recurrent premenstrual tension states of rather severe degree. Although her husband had established the correlation for her between the appearance of these symptoms and the oncoming menstrual period, she nevertheless has always been aware that there was more to it than could be explained by the natural physiological phenomena. When she blurts out that her head feels "like somebody is pushing on it," she makes known to me that her somatic symptoms have incorporated symbolically and have become inseparable from a chronic conflict situation that has to do with other people. Hence, for her to know that it is only a somewhat common premenstrual complaint gives her no comfort. In fact, there is hidden in her symptoms a rather severe depressive state that restates her feelings of helplessness and hopelessness.*)

Dr.: You know, I am particularly interested in what you told me about the pain in the back—in your head—the sense of pressure and the feeling that something is pushing.

Pt.: It's gone now . . .

Dr.: So you feel better now.

Pt.: I can feel myself quiet down when it leaves.

Dr.: Are you warm?

Pt.: A little bit. Just too lazy to take my coat off. (*Patient had come in with her coat on and for the first time had kept it on throughout the interview.*)

Dr.: What do you mean, too lazy?

Pt.: I was busy with this when I came in.

Dr.: And you didn't want to come anyway.

Pt.: No, because I didn't feel good.

Dr.: Any other reason?

Pt.: No. Like last week I felt so good, and this week I said I'm getting discouraged. I don't think I can get better. My husband says, "You are going." He made me come.

Dr.: If it was up to you—

Pt.: I would have stayed home and sat there and felt like this. I felt that let down. My husband couldn't understand why I gave in so fast. I haven't felt so good for so long—and then all of a sudden—it's just like teasing the child with a piece of candy. So I don't know what to think now.

Dr.: How does a child feel who is teased?

Pt.: You give a child a piece of candy, and you take it away—he is resentful when it's gone. That's how I felt.

Dr.: So all your good feeling was gone.

Pt.: Everything was going down the drain.

Dr.: And you felt resentful. Toward whom?

Pt.: Myself, I think—to think that I couldn't keep it up.

Dr.: Do you always blame yourself?

Pt.: Well, there is nobody else I could blame.

Dr.: No?

Pt.: I mean these feelings. I could see it if somebody gets me upset. But when I just get like this. I get angry with myself, and that doesn't help—build things up again.

Dr.: No one else you might be resentful toward. And here you are. You were feeling so much better, and all of a sudden—wham—it's all back again.

Pt.: Like I said to my husband, unless things in my subconscious mind can bother me when I am in my bedroom sleeping—

Dr.: Well, that's certainly possible. You say that when something like this happens, it's like offering a child a piece of candy, and when she reaches for it, it is taken away.

Pt.: That's how I felt.

Dr.: And you feel resentful.

Pt.: Well, that's how I felt.

Dr.: Resentful.

Pt.: I woke up and found myself back where I started.

Dr.: And there are a couple of people you can blame. One is you, and you are used to doing that.

Pt.: Yeah. And I got upset with my son, too, but I didn't get emotional or hurt. I just tried to forget about it. Now whether that stayed in the back of my mind or not—

Dr.: Anyone else you can blame?

Pt.: I don't know.

Dr.: How about your doctor?

Pt.: No, there is only so much that you can do. Then I have to help myself.

Dr.: Maybe, but still—

Pt.: No, I don't think so. I don't see how I can blame you.

Dr.: Well, what do you go to a doctor for?

Pt.: To be helped.

Dr.: And if you are not helped?

Pt.: I feel all right when I am here while I am talking, so I feel that I must be getting some help.

Dr.: Yes, but what happens when you go home?

Pt.: When I go home? Evidently I just let things get a hold of me.

Dr.: It was last week. And before that you were feeling pretty good.

Pt.: I was feeling good.

Dr.: It was last week that things fell apart.

Pt.: Sunday. Saturday. Sunday.

Dr.: Do you think that it might have anything to do with what you and I were talking about last week?

Pt.: You mean, after I left here if it would bother me? No, because I still felt good after I left here. I went shopping and went out that night with my husband shopping, and I went shopping by myself Saturday.

Dr.: Good . . . So when it came, it was kind of a double blow because you were doing so very well.

Pt.: That's how I felt.

Dr.: Yes, but you know, sometimes there are certain experiences that you have that you don't react to till a day later, two days later, sometimes even a week later, and suddenly it hits us . . . Now then, we can go back to my question. Do you remember anything that we talked about last week?

Pt.: I remembered before I came out. I remembered everything before I came out, and now my mind is a—

Dr.: Before you came out. Meaning before you came here today. You mean that you had it kind of rehearsed?

Pt.: No, I was getting ready to come, and I was just thinking. We talked about my father last week.

Dr.: Yes we did.

Pt.: No, my mind is a blank.

Dr.: Is it really?

Pt.: I can't—seem to think back that far now.

Dr.: Anything occur to you, or can't you think of a darn thing?

Pt.: I know that we talked about my father, and I think that we talked about my mother, too.

Dr.: What did we talk about your father?

Pt.: About him going out for his—his entertainment and how he drank heavy—and he seemed happier outside than at home.

Dr.: He felt freer outside than at home.

Pt.: That's all. I could probably think of something that happened twenty years ago, and I can't remember last week.

Dr.: This is not an examination. I am not looking for you to give me the right answer or otherwise you get a zero.

Pt.: No, I am trying to think. I just can't.

Dr.: But we did talk about your father and how he had to leave the house in order to have fun, and outside the house he felt free.

Pt.: Right.

Dr.: Inside?

Pt.: He couldn't get anything he wanted inside.

Dr.: He was not free to do as he pleased inside the house.

Pt.: No, yet he could be boisterous, you know. He was different when he was out. That's all I can remember talking about. Is there something else I should have remembered?

Dr.: If you don't remember there is probably a very good reason. You know that some of these things are not easy to remember, and other things are painful to remember, or sometimes even embarrassing to remember.

Pt.: It can't be painful or embarrassing. I talked about it last week, I should be able to talk about it this week.

Dr.: Well, it's hard to say. For example, I remember something that we talked about last week that you were brave enough to say.

Pt.: That I would rather not come?

Dr.: Yes.

Pt.: Oh, but I came.

SIXTH INTERVIEW

Dr.: Yeah, your husband made you come, didn't he?

Pt.: Last week?

Dr.: This week.

Pt.: Today. Last week I came on my own, but today he made me come.

Dr.: But it was last week—remember what you said about that?

Pt.: I would rather be going shopping or doing something else for enjoyment.

Dr.: Which is perfectly understandable. And I said something to the effect that you were becoming a free citizen. And that meant you are free outside of here, but not here.

Pt.: I am not even half free now this week.

Dr.: This week, yeah.

Pt.: I should be able to accept that we have our ups and downs, but like I said, it felt so good to feel the way I felt last week—was hard to accept this back again.

Dr.: That's true, but do you remember last week you said something about— when you said you were only half free, obviously the other half was if you didn't have to come to see me. Right?

Pt.: Well, I—yeah, that's right.

Dr.: You said that it took courage to say that because you didn't want to hurt me.

Pt.: Mmmm.

Dr.: Do you remember that?

Pt.: Mmmm. Now that you refresh my memory, I remember that.

Dr.: I wonder if this has bothered you since.

Pt.: Because I said that last week? No, no. I went home and told my husband that I told you. So he says, "Well, it's all right." I said, "That's all right because you didn't say it. But that's how I felt, and I felt I had to say it."

Dr.: You told it to him, and he said, "That's okay." And you said, "Yeah, you can say that because you didn't have to say it."

Pt.: Like he says, I spoke how I felt.

Dr.: Yeah.

Pt.: Which I don't ordinarily do.

Dr.: And it took courage on your part. You didn't think that he really fully appreciated how much courage it took for you to say it.

Pt.: No, he said that was good.

Dr.: What did you say?

Pt.: He said, "It was good that you spoke when you told the doctor how you felt." But then I said, "Well, that's all right. It's easy for you to say it's good, but I had"—

Dr.: You are the one who had to say it.

Pt.: Yes, it's not him. It's me, so I have to say it myself.

Dr.: You're the one who had to say it to me—that you would just as soon be rid of me.

Pt.: No, I didn't put it that way.

Dr.: No, I am putting it that way.

Pt.: I don't feel that way. I wish I didn't have to come in. My husband made me come today, but maybe deep down I would have come anyway because I know I am going to get the help—especially where I felt so bad today. I think in the end I would have given in and come.

Dr.: You always give in.

Pt.: I hope that I won't have to give in for too many months. Do you mean that I will always have to come back?

Dr.: Is that the way you feel—that you will always have to come back?

Pt.: I thought that's what you meant—that I wouldn't be all right—that I would always have to give in and come back. (*A remarkably concise, living statement of attachment based upon unresolved ambivalence: "give in and come back."*)

Dr.: Give in and come back?

Pt.: Yeah.

Dr.: Where?

Pt.: To the hospital. I would have to keep coming forever. I don't know if I am going to need that much help. It's getting discouraging to think that I was doing so good and now I am back in the rut again. Maybe I will feel all right next week, I don't know.

Dr.: But this makes you wonder whether you might have to come back and back and back.

Pt.: Mmmm. It makes me think, and like I said to my husband, I am tired of thinking.

Dr.: Let me ask you, how many times have you been here now, seeing me?

Pt.: I think this is the sixth.

Dr.: Huh?

Pt.: I think this is the sixth visit. Sixth or seventh.

Dr.: You kept track?

Pt.: No.

Dr.: So you think it's the sixth or the seventh.

Pt.: Mmmmm.

Dr.: How many do we have?

Pt.: Twelve.

Dr.: So if it's the sixth or the seventh, does that mean anything?

Pt.: Well, to me that means that I am halfway through, and I feel I should be a lot better than I am. I don't know. Sometimes I think that I am doing something wrong somewhere along the line.

Dr.: That you are—

Pt.: That I am not getting better. If I am getting help, I should be getting better.

Dr.: Yes. But then you begin to think that maybe *you* are doing something wrong.

Pt.: Maybe I am not doing everything I am supposed to do.

Dr.: Maybe you are doing everything you are *supposed* to do?

Pt.: And yet I haven't been told what I am supposed to do.

Dr.: That's right.

Pt.: So it's hard to know.

Dr.: You feel a great obligation and need to do what you think I want you to do, don't you?

Pt.: Mmmm. Should I?

Dr.: Should you?

Pt.: I think so. I mean, if you are going for treatments or something, if the doctor tells you to do something, you should do it.

Dr.: What have I told you to do?

Pt.: Nothing except not to take the tranquilizers.

Dr.: Yes, but other than that I haven't told you anything, have I?

Pt.: No. You have never come right out and said, "Don't do this," or "Don't do that."

Dr.: That's right. So how can you feel that you are not doing what I want you to do when I haven't told you what to do?

Pt.: Maybe because when you talk about something and you tell me the cause—that's like saying no to somebody. You said that I had a hard time because I don't say no. So then if I said yes to somebody, well then I say maybe I did wrong.

Dr.: I see what you mean. If I say that you have a hard time saying no—

Pt.: So if I don't say no—

Dr.: Then you think I want you to be able to say no.

Pt.: That's right.

Dr.: So you try to please—

Pt.: I either try to please you or I am misunderstanding what we are talking about.

Dr.: I think that's true, too. But the more important thing is, and you will know better than I, that you like very much to please me.

Pt.: If I am pleasing you, then I know I am helping myself.

Dr.: Let's take the first point. Do you think that it is so that you really want to please me, or is it not so?

Pt.: I can't put it that way.

Dr.: All right.

Pt.: It's like when you told me not to take the pills. I did that—it wasn't exactly to please you. I did it because you told me, and I figured it was for my good, so I didn't take them. It would be easy enough to take them if I had them.

Dr.: Right, but I didn't tell you to say no to somebody. I did not tell you not to take the pills. But when I said that you had a hard time saying no, you took that to mean that I wanted you to say no to somebody.

Pt.: That would be more or less to help myself.

Dr.: That would be, if you would do what you think I want you to do, then that would be helpful to you even if you didn't want to do it.

Pt.: It's hard when you don't want to do it.

Dr.: Then you do have the feeling that you have to do what you think I want you to do.

Pt.: I think so. It's hard to explain.

Dr.: Yes, it is.

Pt.: It's like, if I wanted to conquer my feelings, then I don't have to do what I know I am supposed to do. And yet different things that have been brought out. You brought them out with our conversation. You pointed it out to me, so that's probably where I—

Dr.: You see, what I am trying to help you with at this point is to figure out with you that when you say that you want to do the things that you are supposed to do to help you, it's that—what you are *supposed* to do. Who is saying it to you? Is it you and you alone, or do you feel somebody is pushing on you and saying, "you are *supposed* to do this, you are *supposed* to do that?"

Pt.: I feel that somebody is in the back of my mind. Somebody is saying—

Dr.: You are *supposed* to—

Pt.: Or if an occasion has come up and I have given in, I will say I know that I shouldn't have and I should have said something different.

Dr.: You are saying, no, you *shouldn't* have?

Pt.: Mmmm.

Dr.: And what are you thinking about at that point when you say you shouldn't have?

Pt.: Instead of saying no to somebody because I am too busy—

Dr.: Then you say to yourself.

Pt.: Then something says, "Now you are supposed to say"—

Dr.: Somebody says—I didn't hear you.

Pt.: In the back of my mind somebody is saying that—

Dr.: Ah, yes. "You are supposed to say"—

Pt.: No, if I want to help myself.

Dr.: Whose voice is that in the back of your mind?

Pt.: I don't know. I am thinking of when I have to—

Dr.: Now, you say that because you think I want you to say that, or is it something you have yourself?

Pt.: That's how I feel. That voice is there saying, "Well, you should have said no and you would be helping yourself," but I didn't.

Dr.: I am pressing on the back of your head, aren't I?

Pt.: In a way. But it doesn't bother me much because to me it's supposed to be helping me. And it was up until this week.

Dr.: So something happened this week.

Pt.: Something must have happened somewhere along the line. Like I say, I can't think.

Dr.: Well, maybe you think I am pushing you too much.

Pt.: No.

Dr.: That voice.

Pt.: No, I don't feel that I am being pushed that much. I don't feel that I am being pushed at all.

Dr.: Except—

Pt.: The only thing that I might have is that I should be doing or saying things that should help me. If I do, like say no, or something like that, maybe I am going to feel better. I don't know.

Dr.: I think that what we have to look into is this feeling that you just expressed—that there are times when there is something you haven't done or said, and this voice in back of your mind says you should have. This must be troublesome.

Pt.: It probably isn't too troublesome because I have always been told—

Dr.: You are absolutely right. You have always been told, and you never liked it.

Pt.: No.

Dr.: And I don't think that you like it coming from me, either.

Pt.: Well, that's for my own good, so I am trying to accept it.

Dr.: It may be for your own good. Still, you reacted in a way that you have always been familiar with. You are being pushed. It's hard for you to feel that you are really doing it for yourself.

Pt.: No, because I do try to do it for myself.

Dr.: I know, but still there is the voice in back of your mind that says, "You should have done this, you should have done that."

Pt.: Mmmm. When I do something out of the ordinary, I do feel much better.

Dr.: You do.

Pt.: And I can see it, but I don't get that feeling too often. Of course, I have done it more since I have been coming here, so I feel that much improved.

Dr.: Until this week.

Pt.: Till this week. And the floor just fell through this week. I hope it doesn't last too long.

Dr.: You know, you said to me last week that you sit here getting to be free—only half free. The other half is not to have to come here.

Pt.: That's right.

Dr.: That took courage on your part to say.

Pt.: Mmmm.

Dr.: What I am suggesting is that perhaps you know that not only did it take courage, you have been a little worried about it—that maybe you didn't say the right thing or the nice thing.

Pt.: Because I said no? That didn't bother me.

Dr.: You felt good about it—about saying it?

Pt.: Well, I expressed how I felt. I felt I had half the load off my shoulders, and the other half was to come. Now I have to get rid of it all over again.

Dr.: But what is the load?

Pt.: Just like I say, we are halfway there now.

Dr.: Half the load is off your shoulders. There is another half to get rid of. But what is the load?

Pt.: Just straighten out and feel good. Stop getting these feelings. I don't know if I can.

Dr.: Don't you feel that I am something of a load to you?

Pt.: No, no. Because I stop and think, what if I didn't come at all.

Dr.: Maybe. Still, do you feel pressured by me?

Pt.: No—no. I don't talk ordinarily at home like this.

Dr.: You don't feel any pressure from me?

Pt.: No—no—I don't think that I do.

Dr.: You don't feel any pressure to please me?

Pt.: No, not pressure. I feel that I should because—

Dr.: You should please me?

Pt.: I should do what I feel you want me to do.

Dr.: There you are again. Now what did I tell you to do?

Pt.: No, not that you told me to do.

Dr.: Is it the things that you—

Pt.: Think.

Dr.: Think. Is it the things that you think I want you to do?

Pt.: Anything we talk about. And if it is something that's been bothering me, then I feel that I should eliminate that because we spoke about it, and then I am going to feel better once I eliminate it.

Dr.: I see. Since we spoke about it, then that should take care of that. And if it doesn't take care of it right away, then you are troubled because you are not doing—

Pt.: What—

Dr.: You think—

Pt.: I think I should be.

Dr.:	What you think you should do in order to please *me* as well.
Pt.:	Well, I figure I will please you if I tell you that I conquered this, or eliminated that.
Dr.:	There it is again. How much are you doing it for me, and how much is it for you?
Pt.:	I don't know. It's confusing.
Dr.:	Yes, but then it has always been so for you.
Pt.:	Maybe I can straighten that out.
Dr.:	Can you believe that you don't have to do to please me?
Pt.:	Oh, I don't have to, because I don't think that there is anything we have mentioned that I had to do.
Dr.:	But that's how you feel. And it's an old feeling of yours.
Pt.:	To please?
Dr.:	Yes. Always. How to please everybody.
Pt.:	I tried.
Dr.:	And you tried to please me. It's natural for you to try to do that.
Pt.:	I have to conquer that. Like I say, anything that we bring out I feel that I am going to have to conquer that.
Dr.:	But there is nothing to conquer. Who shall you please, you or me?
Pt.:	Myself.
Dr.:	That's right. You don't have to please me one bit.
Pt.:	No, but if I did something that you thought I shouldn't have—and I figure, well, why am I coming here if I am not going to do what I think is right by you.
Dr.:	And if you don't do what you think I want you to, then you come in and tell me, and I will say, "Now look here, toe the line or get out."
Pt.:	Well, then you will ask me why am I coming.
Dr.:	Yes. If you don't listen to me, then why are you coming?
Pt.:	That's how I feel.
Dr.:	But you don't have to do what you think I want you to do.
Pt.:	You're getting me confused again.
Dr.:	I know that it's hard for you to separate the two. It's hard for you to feel entirely free.
Pt.:	Right. I should have hung around Abraham Lincoln. Maybe he could have freed me. I have felt it, but I am getting discouraged.
Dr.:	Sure you are.
Pt.:	It's hard enough not to say it—and I can't lie about it—but like today when I feel that I haven't conquered anything.
Dr.:	Who says you have to?
Pt.:	I feel that I shouldn't be wasting your time. I should feel better now.
Dr.:	Who says you are wasting my time?
Pt.:	I am, I guess.
Dr.:	Did I say it?
Pt.:	No.
Dr.:	No. Did I say you had to conquer anything that we talk about?
Pt.:	No. It's all misunderstood.
Dr.:	Don't blame yourself for it. You are reacting and feeling this way all your life. You know that voice in back of your mind?
Pt.:	My mother?

Dr.: Yes, except that I am there, too, now.

Pt.: So I have an addition. No wonder my poor head feels like somebody is pushing me.

Dr.: That's right.

Pt.: So how is this stopping me from sleeping, though—always get back to that because it's an awful problem. If I knew what to do—I mean, in this case now I look for answers.

Dr.: I know. You want me to tell you what to do. I am not going to, because everybody tells you what to do.

Pt.: I am not looking for you to tell me what to do. I am looking for advice.

Dr.: Same thing for you. You know, you just said something that is very important for you. This voice in back of your mind, pressing—yes, your mother, me, people telling you what to do and when to do—it makes anyone resentful. You said yourself it's like a kid offered a piece of candy and then it is pulled away. Of course, I think that you feel resentful, too.

Pt.: I do. I don't know if it's resentment or sometimes just plain angry when I don't feel good. I wasn't one to get angry.

Dr.: You are allowed, you know, to have angry feelings.

Pt.: I can see getting angry with someone, but not over you.

Dr.: You are allowed to be angry about me, too.

Pt.: If you said something, I don't know if I could get angry.

Dr.: I am not ordering you to get angry, or saying that you have to get angry to please me. I am saying that this pressure in back of your head, I think you feel comes as much from me—that you are supposed to be doing—

Pt.: Is this going to hurt me more than help me if I keep on thinking this way—as far as getting treated?

Dr.: Again, you see, if I tell you and give you the answers, you will say now you know what to do. Do you know what I mean?

Pt.: What I mean is it going to affect me in any way, because I come home and take the same attitude toward my mother or somebody as with you?

Dr.: You will have to learn to be yourself. You don't have to do what I say, or even try to figure out what I am trying to say so that you can do it—but to feel simply free, as free as you can to do whatever you feel.

Pt.: I can try. But I will have to. It's like a job. I have to keep pushing myself at it.

Dr.: Well, that is the difference between if you push yourself or you feel you are being pushed, and this—

Pt.: Is being pushed.

Dr.: Yes, someone is pushing you. You feel this pressure on your head as though someone or something is pushing you.

Pt.: I still don't see why I have been waking up like that every night.

Dr.: I am not clear about that yet either. We can learn more about that.

Pt.: I hope so.

Dr.: How is your head now?

Pt.: It's all right now.

Dr.: You feel a little more alive.

Pt.: I feel I can go home now and go on the bus. I don't think I need a cab.

Dr.: I will see you next week.

Pt.: Yes.

*As we come to the midpoint of the twelve interviews, we find that
the patient keeps accurate account of the number. All of her ambivalence in respect to separation pours out. All the progress—she had
felt the best in more than ten years—collapses and disappears in the
course of the week. She feels so awful and so discouraged as to wonder whether she will have to come back (to the therapist) forever.
This is a beautiful expression of the unconscious wish to cling to the
unresolved ambivalence instead of daring the fear and pain of an
effective separation. The kind of relationship she has had and continues to have with her mother is well revealed in the bursting pressure
in her head and in the voice in back of her mind. Can she risk the
murderous resentment which would have to be faced were she to
decide on separating herself from both the real mother and the intro-
jected mother in their controlling aspects? Can she conquer mother?
At the midpoint of treatment, these doubts become manifest in a
flagrant renewal of symptoms, with particular emphasis on a host of
anxiety symptoms along with persistent insomnia. She seems to have
little inclination to give up her newfound freedom in respect to
going out alone, however, and this is a favorable prognostic indication
because it speaks for the strength of her wish to be free.*

*Understanding the negative transference concealed in the rush of
symptoms and in the discouragement of the patient, and cognizant of
its being the midpoint, I was not hesitant in pressing the patient to
recognize, or to feel, that I, too, am her tormentor. The repetitious-
ness of much of the interview arises because it was necessary to
clarify and to elaborate over and over again the patient's life style so
that it might be possible for her to begin to feel me as her tormentor,
rather than to surrender to such a statement by me in line with her
practically automatic need to please. The uphill battle toward termination will soon be under way.*

*Much of the latter half of the interview is also repetitious. It illus-
trates the kind of convoluted, obsessional thinking upon which much
psychotherapy of any kind founders. In this instance, every effort is
made to diminish the isolation of affect characteristic of this neurotic
disorder by insistently bringing the central issue in its relation to me.
The patient is deeply disappointed in me. We have come to the halfway mark, she had gotten rid of half her load, and suddenly everything crumbles. I make no effort to turn aside her disappointment
but press on toward her privilege of allowing her feelings about me
to come into the open.*

Seventh Interview

*She is feeling somewhat better once more and has continued to go
out alone. She has had a cold, her children are taking turns with the*

*flu which has kept her well occupied. She has tried something new
in her effort to overcome her continuing insomnia. She has left the
bedroom she shares with her husband and has taken to sleeping alone
on a downstairs couch. Since she has thus separated herself so as not
to disturb her husband's sleep, I suggest that we now look closely
into what it is that keeps her from sleeping.*

Dr.: Let's talk about this problem. When you go to bed and you don't sleep, what happens?

Pt.: I fall asleep, but then I wake up.

Dr.: And when you get up, what happens—jittery did you say? What is that like?

Pt.: I am nervous. I get the hot feeling, the hot flash, and my head gets hot and starts pounding. It goes away and then it comes back again. It keeps going on until I get completely exhausted and I fall asleep again.

Dr.: Your heart will pound, and you will get hot.

Pt.: I wake up and I am soaked and wet and perspiring.

Dr.: Is there anything that happens to wake you up?

Pt.: I have these thoughts or nightmares. Nine times out of ten it will be that something happened to the children. Lately, since my mother has been sick, it's something happening to her. That's why I don't like to go to bed, because it's either a nightmare or I wake up like that, so I wait till I am completely exhausted. It's not really good because I am not getting proper rest.

Dr.: You say that one of the things that makes you not like to go to bed is that you are afraid that you are going to have these nightmares—something terrible happens to the children or something to your mother. What might you dream about your mother?

Pt.: Oh, a couple of times I dreamt that she was dying . . . I dream she is suffering. She is in pain, and when I wake up I am all nervous and perspiring . . .

Dr.: Does this jitteriness, palpitation, feeling so hot and perspired only happen at night?

Pt.: Most of the time. Maybe during the day if something happens that upsets me—the children get hurt or something. They would have to fall and I would have to see blood before it would excite me that much. They are always falling and getting hurt.

Dr.: Tell me, some people go to bed and fall asleep quickly, but lots of people, at one time or another, lie in bed for a while and think various things. Are you the kind of person who lies in bed and thinks about different things?

Pt.: I go to bed and try not to, but—but it manages to creep in my mind.

Dr.: What kind of things creep in your mind?

Pt.: It's usually the security of the children. I will be laying there and I will be thinking—you hear about all these fires and different things like that. It's—

Dr.: Kind of frightening things?

Pt.: Yes, I think of them out playing, and something happens—

Dr.: Out playing and what?

Pt.: Out playing during the day, and what if something happens to them—They fall and get hurt. Like if I have read the paper or heard on the news.

Dr.: When you go to bed, one of the things that is apt to happen as you are

THE CASE OF THE CONQUERED WOMAN

lying there—you begin to think about the security of the children: fires, what might have happened while they were playing today, what might happen tomorrow. You must scare the hell out of yourself.

Pt.: More or less. I am usually looking for an answer of how can I protect them so that things won't happen. It's foolish, because what happens is going to happen. But I can't make myself understand that. I understand it, but I can't make myself let it go at that.

For the first time she is able to enter with me into her more secret, calamitous mind. Here all her angry badness lies. Something terrible will happen to her children; her mother is dying. She searches desperately for ways to protect her children from tragedy. She adds that she did not dwell so on tragedy until her own children came along, nor had she any difficulty sleeping until they came. The children respond to her constant cautions about danger by unconsciously addressing themselves to mother's unconscious when they say to her, "Stop telling us to be careful. You jinx us." In school, when they are playing in the street, at the beach, or alone in the house, the children are never safe in her mind. She avoids watching violence on television. Her mother was never this way, and yet she finds herself obsessionally trapped in the expectation of tragedy befalling her children.

We learn that she has a particularly morbid fear of fire, and that this began when she was twelve years old. She often babysat for her sister's six-year-old boy when his mother went out to do her shopping on Saturday afternoons. On one occasion, the patient had gone to an afternoon movie, and a neighbor had been asked to keep an eye on the boy. That day the boy's trousers caught fire while he was playing with matches with other boys in the street. The patient was called out of the movie and told what had happened, and she accompanied the boy to the hospital. After lingering for two years, he succumbed to the complications of the burns. Although it is evident that she had no responsibility for what had happened, as an already guilt-laden child, she promptly absorbed the whole incident. The guilty horror of it has ever since evoked horrified fascination with calamity.

Dr.: So, fire is one of the tragedies that—
Pt.: I would say the main one . . .
Dr.: You know that some people who are always thinking about automobile accidents, or fires, or things like that—while it is frightening for them to think about, yet these things interest them, too. You know, a kind of frightened fascination.
Pt.: No. I know what you are getting at. No.
Dr.: What am I getting at?
Pt.: Something like—even start a fire and enjoy it.
Dr.: You are way ahead of me. I wasn't for one moment thinking of you start-

ing a fire, but what I am saying is that sometimes a person who is always worried about something happening, in a kind of strange way perhaps is fascinated by that very same terrible thing.

Pt.: You mean they could stand there and be fascinated?

Dr.: Oh, no. Just the thought. You see, one of the things that does bother you is that when you think something, you are the kind of person who has the understanding and the feeling that whatever you think is the same as something really happening. Do you follow me?

Pt.: Actually it's happening in me . . .

Dr.: There are two things mainly. One is when you go to bed, one of the things that does keep you up is that you find that your mind quickly gets to thinking these terrible thoughts. The other thing is that when you think these terrible thoughts, it becomes very real for you, so that when you think about what might happen to your children, it becomes so real that you scare yourself out of your wits.

Pt.: If that's happening, why can't I correct it?

Dr.: I think that you can. First of all, you have to—I don't know if you ever thought about it in this way, that you may be the kind of person who thinks that whatever she thinks is the same as the deed. When you think about something happening to your children, you react as though something really happened . . .

Pt.: I never thought of it that way . . .

Dr.: What kind of rating do you give yourself?

Pt.: I feel that I am a good person. I probably could be better if I weren't to dwell on these things and give me a better disposition.

Dr.: What's that?

Pt.: I feel that I am a good person, but with a bad disposition.

Dr.: A bad disposition?

Pt.: When I am nervous and unhappy—and worrying.

Dr.: Because of these terrible frightening thoughts about your children, and now about your mother too. When you think them they are very real to you, as though it happened.

Pt.: It seems as if everything does happen. I feel I have already gone through that before.

Dr.: Oh, a hundred times.

Pt.: And I have often wanted to go back.

Dr.: Say that again.

Pt.: If something happens, or I go someplace, I feel that I have already been there, or it has already happened.

Dr.: For example—

Pt.: It doesn't necessarily have to be anything bad either. Like I say, I went to a party or a wedding.

Dr.: You feel that you have been there?

Pt.: I feel I have been there.

Dr.: What do you think about that?

Pt.: I don't know. I have often thought about it.

Dr.: Think that you are crazy?

Pt.: I don't know what the significance of it was. Somebody came into the house, and I would feel like I have already had them come in and entertained them before. Like if the children fall and get cut, I will say I knew that would happen. Maybe it's like you explained to me, I think these things—maybe I dwell so much on them that it is real, and I feel like it has happened to me before. (*I do believe that what she has been describing are not déjà vu experiences. Rather, stimulated by my explanation of the magical quality of her thinking, she then reveals how pervasive this is. She has undoubtedly thought about weddings and parties and entertaining certain people. When these actually occur, she feels she has already been through them—and she has, in her thoughts.*)

Dr.: You are one of those people that whatever you think becomes the same to you as though it were real, actual, as though it happened.

Pt.: It seems rather odd. If you have never been there, why should you feel you have been there? I go to a strange place, and you know just where everything is . . .

Dr.: You mean you have been in a pretty strange place, and you have known where everything was?

Pt.: Possibly I could have dreamt it or something. I wouldn't say I knew where the rooms were, or this or that, but I would get there—

Dr.: I don't know about that, but I do know that a person like yourself who dwells so much on terrible things happening is the kind of person who also feels that just to think it makes it so. (*I return to my contention about her mode of thinking because it is too important to let it get lost. She is deeply concerned about her magical thinking which is intensified by the confusion arising in her mind between thoughts occurring during the day, thoughts while lying awake in bed, and dreams and nightmares. Thus, she suggests that it may relate to dreams. There was never anything to be observed clinically to suggest loss of reality or threatened reality loss.*)

Pt.: Makes it real.

Dr.: Just because you think something, then it is so. When you think about something terrible happening to your children, it is as though it were real.

Pt.: Really happening.

Dr.: Right. So you get all in a tizzy, because for you it is real.

Pt.: That could be possible because just worrying certainly shouldn't make me the way I am so now. I am just a worrier.

Dr.: You are not a normal worrier, you worry more than normal.

Pt.: I will have to learn to stop worrying. It's very hard to go from one extreme to another.

Dr.: There is not much danger.

Pt.: Well, they do need protection till they are old enough to be on their own, too.

Dr.: Do you think that you might go from one extreme all the way to the other?

Pt.: I don't know. I am saying it might be possible. I hope it isn't. I wouldn't want to leave them without any protection . . . (*The characteristic fear of the obsessional—that the resolution of total restraint can only lead to total release.*)

Dr.: I am sure that they don't want you with them all the time.

Pt.: No, not even the little one. They like to be on their own.

Dr.: You know, this is another thing that contributes to your general sense of dissatisfaction and unhappiness. You find yourself so often having these calamitous, tragic thoughts about people who are very close and very important to you, and you drive yourself into a tizzy.

Pt.: I just dwell on it.

Dr.: That's how you drive yourself into a tizzy. As you think about it, it becomes so real that you get all wound up, and the more you convince yourself of how real this is—

Pt.: The worse I get.

Dr.: And you worry still more. Just as you told me, you lie in bed and think about what might have happened yesterday. And that's not enough, so you start working on what might happen tomorrow. Then it all becomes real, and you start to shake—jump out of bed or whatever. You can't sleep.

Pt.: No, I can't sleep when I start that.

Dr.: Where are you going now?

Pt.: Home. I think my daughter has enough—

Dr.: Are you going to see how many calamities occurred?

Pt.: No. I will go home and try to doctor my son, who says he isn't sick.

In exploring her night problem, the patient begins to reveal the nature of her phobic behavior and the overprotective behavior she imposes on her children. Tragedies and calamities, fires and accidents— all the terrible things that could have happened yesterday or will surely happen tomorrow. We learn for the first time something about her feelings of guilt in connection with failure to fulfill whatever responsibility is asked of her, and we get some clues about the combination of aggressive fantasies and the guilt accompanying them being intensified by an accident of reality, which contributes to the further growth and impact of magical thinking in an open way into her adult life. Bad thoughts assure that bad events will happen. No wonder it becomes imperative for her to be "good," compliant, and to please. The consequences of any other kind of behavior are too horrible to contemplate. As we pass the midpoint of treatment, the kind of unconscious conflicts that perpetuate attachment and failure of individuation becomes available for the work of treatment. Until this point, insomnia has remained vague as to its cause. Now we hear of nightmarish aggressive and destructive fantasies that can be prevented from becoming real only by remaining closely attached to the objects in jeopardy.

Eighth Interview

The patient called in to say that she was ill and would not be in for her regular appointment. She would come the following week.

All was well with the patient until the day before the appointment, when she found that she had some abscessed teeth. She was able to ask very comfortably that I end the interview a few minutes early so that she could make her appointment with the dentist. She reported that she had had one "bad night" during the preceding week. Recall-

ing that she had felt similarly just one month before, she made the connection with her menses, and significantly, her distress promptly came to an end. She has been sleeping well and has made an entirely new sleeping arrangement in the family. Her husband now sleeps with her on a new couch downstairs, so that both are away from the bedrooms of the children. Now she sleeps well and has begun to eat well, perhaps too well. At one point, I noted that she was scratching her arms. To my inquiry she said that she has been breaking out mildly at times ever since the original episode of hives. She is apt to become itchy whenever she is unduly warm. "I was like that down at my mother's. After I had done her work I was very warm and I started to itch and to break out." She did not wish to do the housework for her mother but did it anyway. Mother surprised the patient by not telling her what to do and even thanked her for doing it. I remarked that the patient had been very good.

Pt.: Which I don't like to keep saying. I am always afraid that I am going to jinx myself—something is going to happen.

Dr.: You are afraid that you are going to jinx yourself?

Pt.: I am used to saying that I don't feel good, that this bothers me. So when I do say that I feel good, it seems odd. But everybody has been noticing that I have been feeling good, too. The children even remarked about it. I seem to have more patience.

Dr.: The children have said to you—haven't they said that you sometimes jinx them?

Pt.: Mmmm. When they are going out the door. So I am learning not to say, "Be careful." I just don't say anything. I just let them go.

Dr.: You control yourself.

Pt.: Yes, and I haven't had any nightmares, either, which we were talking about. I figured if that was bothering me, I would have to buckle down and try to get it out of my head, and it has been working.

Dr.: Let me ask you something in that connection. Do you remember the last time you were here, we were talking about these terrible thoughts you were getting in your head at night, and all kinds of terrible things happening, especially to the kids. This was one reason why when they would go out, you would tell them to be careful, and they would say that you will jinx them. Then you told me something that I have been wondering about ever since. I wanted to check it with you. You told me about your sister's boy.

Pt.: The one that got burned? . . . *(Here I take the opportunity to learn more, if possible, about this terrible episode, which came during the patient's early adolescent years. Not much more is obtained except that the patient told how she put the whole thing out of her mind after the boy died. So far as she was concerned, the incident had been removed from her awareness. However, she continued to say that although all concern about the event quieted down after he died, "I never seemed to think about him except when I hear of children playing with matches, or I see my children going too near the stove.")*

Dr.: Near the stove. You mean in your house?

Pt.: Yeah. Like the older ones. I always say, "Be careful," or if I see them grab a book of matches, I always take it away, and I proceed to tell them what happened to my nephew.

Dr.: You do tell them? What do you tell?

Pt.: That he had been burnt because the boys were playing with fire and that he died. I don't go into extremes with it, but I don't think it registers with the children because they always seem to—look at matches, and we have to keep watching. Not that I ever caught them playing with matches . . .

Dr.: Did it ever occur to you—did you ever find yourself wondering or thinking that, on that particular day you decided to go to the movies, what would have happened if you had not decided to go the movies?

Pt.: I would have been babysitting, and when I did that I kept the children in the house. They didn't go out. I would keep them in the house where I could watch them.

Dr.: Then if you had been babysitting, would this have happened?

Pt.: It could have happened in the house, I suppose. If things are going to happen they are going to happen.

Dr.: If you were babysitting that day, would he have been outside?

Pt.: No. She always kept the children in the house when I babysat.

Dr.: Do you know what I am getting at?

Pt.: If I babysat I would have prevented it.

Dr.: I have wondered if you had this in your mind, that if you hadn't been—

Pt.: At the movies.

Dr.: At the movies, maybe this might not have happened—therefore, whether you have always felt a little bit guilty yourself about it.

Pt.: I don't even remember thinking about feeling guilty or blaming myself. I mean, if it were a case if she had asked me to babysit, and I said no—

Dr.: I see. But this helps me to understand why you are so careful.

Pt.: It's just a deep fear of fire in me.

Dr.: And why you would be so frightened about your children, and watch over them, perhaps too closely.

Pt.: Probably. I mean, I didn't see him on fire, but I saw his body and it always stays in my mind. Even today, if I see children on the street with matches, I will get off the bus and stop them.

Dr.: Really?

Pt.: Probably get picked up someday for not minding my own business, but I just can't walk by—I can't see children playing with matches or fire.

Dr.: You have never forgotten that.

Pt.: No. It was the same time as the Coconut Grove fire, and all the talk about that. There were people in the hospital at the same time as my nephew.

Dr.: From the Coconut Grove fire?

Pt.: They had come there. So there was a lot there that stayed in my mind. I had the fear of fire, but I never felt guilty about it . . .

Dr.: Now we can understand to this day—fire and kids playing with matches.

Pt.: It's an awful fear with me.

Dr.: Now let's look at it in another way. Your kids. Say they are going out, and you say, "Be careful." They say, "Don't jinx us." What do they mean?

Pt.: I don't know. I suppose if they fall, they say that's because I said be careful . . .

Dr.: It's possible by always telling kids to be careful, be careful, be careful, you kind of remind them not to be careful.

Pt.: I don't know. I suppose I keep saying, "Be careful," so much, maybe they think they don't have to be so careful.

Dr.: Yes.

Pt.: And they just go out. That's children—they don't stop to think. If they had to think all day long, it wouldn't be any fun going out and playing.

Dr.: That's right. Now as far as you are concerned, though, you are somewhat hesitant to say that you have been feeling good because you don't want to jinx yourself.

Pt.: Well, I'm always saying that I don't feel good, I have this wrong or that wrong. It's been good for two weeks. Even when I had the flu I felt good, which is not common to feel good when you are sick. But like I said to my husband, it felt good to be sick and yet not nervous about anything. And I got over that and I had a nice holiday. I wasn't nervous, and I enjoyed cooking the meals for them, and the children played, and I didn't have to speak up to them or anything. Whereas ordinarily I would be yelling, "Pick this up," or "Do this." And I just let them go and play.

Dr.: So you have been very good.

Pt.: I noticed they haven't bothered me too much. I think I kind of made up my mind. I am not going to let them aggravate me, and if they messed up things, they can pick it up later, and it will get done eventually. So from one day to the next I tried to cope with things, and it has been working so far.

Dr.: How do you figure it all out?

Pt.: I think I am facing things more openly. If the children do something wrong, I will stop and think about what I am going to reprimand them about and if it makes any sense, or if it's just better to forget what they have done because it isn't that important. I try to question myself before I go any further, and when I go to bed at night, I don't say that I am not going to sleep. I say I am going to sleep. I try that psychology . . .

Dr.: How do you feel inside you?

Pt.: I feel calm, more calm than I felt for a long time. My stomach isn't jumpy, and I have been eating. Like I say, I just feel good. I don't know. It's hard to explain.

Dr.: You are willing to accept it as it is.

Pt.: I don't question it. I just want to stay this way. I don't have to question it. I know why I feel better—because I am trying to face facts. Instead of pushing them in the back of my mind, I bring them out and—

Dr.: Facts like what?

Pt.: I mean like whatever bothers me. I get to the bottom of it. If the children have done something that really bothers me, then we talk about it.

Dr.: You talk about it with the—

Pt.: With the children. I don't wait for my husband to come home at night. I settle it with them myself.

Dr.: You aren't holding it in and making believe it doesn't bother you. Is that what you mean?

Pt.: I get rid of it right then and there—whatever they do.

Dr.: And how are things between you and your husband?

Pt.: They have been good.

Dr.: What does he say to all this?

Pt.: He thinks it's fine, and he can see an improvement, except like last Saturday. Like I said, I didn't feel good, and he remarked about that.

Dr.: Was that before your period?

Pt.: It's usually about a week before. And then Monday, I was very cranky with the children with everything. And that passed, you know. That was the only time. I didn't have any pressure with my head like I did last time. I haven't had that for over a month now.

Dr.: This was last Saturday night. Tell me, what it is that you had on Saturday night?

Pt.: I just felt nervous and jumpy.

Dr.: Hot feelings?

Pt.: No, not so much the hot feeling—the upset feeling.

Dr.: What Saturday night was that?

Pt.: I think it was after I came home from my mother's. But of course, when I come home from my mother's, I discovered my daughter had chicken pox. I might have just gotten upset over that.

Dr.: If it isn't one thing, it's five other things.

Pt.: I just thought of that.

Dr.: That she has chicken pox?

Pt.: Mmmm, and that didn't bother me.

Dr.: I suppose it didn't bother you because it's not a serious thing. But it is another burden.

Pt.: She wasn't too bad. It wasn't too much of a burden. She was really itchy, but she wasn't sick.

Dr.: You came home after doing your mother's—

Pt.: Doing the housework. She greeted me at the door, "Look at me." So I looked and I said, "That's nice, so go to bed."

Dr.: She said, "Look at me," and you looked and you said, "That's nice, go to bed." Do you remember what you felt?

Pt.: I just felt like everything collapsing on me. And I thought she would be sick because my other children when they had it were sick.

Dr.: Okay now. I know that you want to get away early today to get to the dentist.

The patient had done very well in a longer interval between visits than had been the case. Note how she always describes her emotional state in terms of good and bad, and how her usual response is that she is "doing good." She is largely symptom-free, is sleeping well, and uses no medications of any kind. It was a mark of progress for her to be able to tell me that she had a dental appointment and that our time would have to be a bit shortened. I explored the burned-child incident at length in order to determine whether she could be helped to see and to feel the affective relationship between that event and her current fear, and to open her guilt so that the tie to that past event could be weakened. She demonstrates how much of the episode she has repressed, but at the same time reveals that the strength of her repression is not so great. When pressed, she does recall and re-member, perhaps more than she wishes to. The point is that I found her to be well defended against the guilt that must be present, with her compensatory overprotectiveness and reaction formation (taking matches away from strange children) serving this purpose very well. She is feeling better and behaving better in many ways. I wonder whether she can go on being good as we approach the termination phase.

Ninth Interview

Dr.: *(Patient arrives several minutes late and out of breath.)* What happened?

Pt.: My husband was rushing home. I had a hard time getting a cab. (Sighs.)

Dr.: Are you worried about being late?

Pt.: I didn't want to be late because I didn't know whether I would just have to go right back home or not.

Dr.: What do you mean?

Pt.: It mean, it's specified 1:15, and I didn't know if I was late you would cancel my appointment.

Dr.: You didn't know whether I would wait?

Pt.: I didn't know. I figured if it was 1:30 or later—

Dr.: It's still your time.

Pt.: Oh.

Dr.: Tell me about you . . . *(She still has some sick children around but con-tinues to feel quite well. She had had a nightmare the night before this visit and feels that it was precipitated by a movie she had been watching on television.)*

Pt.: I woke up perspiring and my heart was pounding. I could see my children falling in a pit. They were getting a drink out of a bubbler, and the ground just sunk. I looked down and they were in water. I could see one on the bottom. My brother happened to be there, and he jumped in and saved her. Then I woke up and I was perspiring. I had been watching a movie about deep-sea diving, so maybe it had something to do with that.

Dr.: You had this nightmare while you were asleep. Now, tell me, were all of the children at the bubbler?

Pt.: No, there were three.

Dr.: The three youngest?

Pt.: The three youngest.

Dr.: The three youngest were at the bubbler getting a drink, and what happened?

Pt.: The bubbler just sunk and they went down, and it seemed to be some kind of basement of some sort. There seemed to be water, and one was swim-ming and trying to save herself. The other one at the bottom was the little boy. It was like an elevator. It was a confused dream but they managed to all get out.

Dr.: They did get out.

Pt.: So when I got up—and prior to that I used to have these nightmares I would wake up my husband and I would be all upset.

Dr.: Not this time?

Pt.: I got up and had a glass of water and went back to bed.

Dr.: Have you ever had a nightmare like this?

Pt.: About the children drowning?

Dr.: This sort of thing.

Pt.: Yeah, a couple of times.

Dr.: Can you recall the last time?

Pt.: The last time was when we had been visiting somebody and my little girl Tammy—she's six, and she was only about two—and she had fallen in their pool. But we were all there so my husband was able to jump in and drag her. After that I kept dreaming—I could see her in the bottom of the pool.

Dr.: That would have been then four years ago. And since then?

Pt.: Not about drowning, no.

Dr.: Nothing like this?

Pt.: No, not that I can recall. Not drowning anyway.

Dr.: Would you like to see if we can figure out what this nightmare might have to do with you?

Pt.: I don't mind. I always figure it was normal to have nightmares. But I didn't think it was normal to have the reactions I had that I couldn't control myself once I woke up.

Dr.: Well, you know that these nightmares have meaning, too, don't they?

Pt.: I suppose they do.

Dr.: I mean, they are not just accidents. They have some meaning. You have told me a million times how you are very protective about your children; you are always afraid that some terrible thing will happen. This time you were watching a picture about—

Pt.: Deep-sea diving.

Dr.: Alone?

Pt.: My husband was asleep, and I was watching.

Dr.: Let's see if I have the events. Your husband went to bed, but you didn't.

Pt.: I sat on the chair and watched for a while. Then I got in bed and tried to watch the rest of it but fell asleep . . .

Dr.: What do you think about that nightmare?

Pt.: It didn't have any significance. I figured I had watched the movie. That's what it was. It was too farfetched about the ground. I think it was—caving in.

Dr.: In a building?

Pt.: A house, or something like a building. It seemed that a lot of people were going over to the bubbler to get a drink. The ground was soft, like it was newly finished, and I kept saying that's going to sink. And some would go down, and they would come up. I said, "Well, I am not going over there because I am not going down." Somebody said, "No, you are not, but your children already went down."

Dr.: And then you said—

Pt.: I could see them.

Dr.: Now who did you see?

Pt.: I saw Tammy. She was at the bottom.

Dr.: What was she doing?

Pt.: She was just laying there. And Jessica was swimming, and Wally was sitting like in a shaft like an elevator, eating something. I don't know. It wasn't bothering him. He was in the water, but it didn't bother him.

Dr.: Sitting in this sort of elevator shaft.

Pt.: When he came up it was the baby, so it was all confused.

Dr.: When he came up it wasn't—

Pt.: It wasn't him, it was the baby.

Dr.: Are you amused by it?

Pt.: It didn't really bother me, which ordinarily it did. I mean, I woke up and I said, "That's crazy," and I just went back to sleep, which was bad since I overslept and then everybody was late.

Dr.: What I am struck by is that you said you were frightened about it.

Pt.: Well, when I woke up about five minutes things run through my mind after that.

Dr.: Can you remember what ran through your mind?

Pt.: I remember that I was trying to realize that it was a dream, and I was waking up. You sit on the edge of the bed and you say, "Well, is it true or isn't it?" And all of a sudden you are awake. Before I used to wake up my husband, and this would go on for hours, but I just couldn't—

Dr.: This time you accepted it yourself as a dream.

Pt.: As a dream, and then I went back to sleep, which is unusual.

Dr.: Now I am going to ask you a very funny question. What about relations with your husband? (*This is my association to some of the elements in her nightmare which suggested the wish for and fear of having a baby.*)

Pt.: Well, in what manner?

Dr.: What do you think I mean?

Pt.: You mean argue?

Dr.: No.

Pt.: We get along. We get along good. There doesn't seem to be any arguments as far as the children are taken care of. And our sex life, we agree on that.

Dr.: What about your sex life. Would you like to tell me about that?

Pt.: There is nothing special with me in regard to it. Other than being a mental patient, I would like more children.

Dr.: Would you?

Pt.: I would but I don't think—

Dr.: Other than being a mental case.

Pt.: Well, the condition I am in and still wanting more. But once the little one starts to walk around, kind of, you know, you would like to see another little one in the crib. But that isn't going over too good.

Dr.: What do you mean?

Pt.: My husband said to forget it. We have enough to handle.

Dr.: What do you do about it?

Pt.: We follow rhythm.

Dr.: Have you always followed rhythm?

Pt.: Mmmm.

Dr.: Has it always worked?

Pt.: It's always worked. I think once—but I don't remember which one it was.

Dr.: It didn't work?

Pt.: It did work, but I was very irregular. I think that was on Wally.

Dr.: Of course, if you are irregular, then you are going to get caught. Are you regular now?

Pt.: Yes.

Dr.: Do you know whether in your cycle you are safe now?

Pt.: What do you mean? Can I time myself?

Dr.: When was the last time you had intercourse, for example.

Pt.: Yesterday.

Dr.: Last night?

Pt.: Mmmm. Now that would be the end of it. I had my period all last week, and then we take the one day after and seven days before.

Dr.: Your period ended when?

Pt.: Wednesday.

Dr.: Day before yesterday.

Pt.: Mmmm. So yesterday—

Dr.: Yesterday, you were safe.

Pt.: Safe. And then seven or eight days before.

Dr.: I thought that you might have had intercourse last night.

Pt.: Why?

Dr.: Because your dream says that.

Pt.: I am going to have nightmares because I—

Dr.: No. You want a baby.

Pt.: Well, I don't know. That's too bad.

Dr.: Maybe. But you really want one.

Pt.: I would like another one.

Dr.: I think that it's important for you to recognize that you do want a baby. Your husband says?

Pt.: He says no. He figures my health is at stake, that's all. He loves the children, too. He is as crazy as I am to have a little one around.

Dr.: So there is a kind of conflict right now between you and your husband on this.

Pt.: I wouldn't call it a conflict.

Dr.: I would.

Pt.: No. I mean, he would like one as well as I would.

Dr.: Yes, but he says no.

Pt.: Well, he has to say no.

Dr.: What do you mean?

Pt.: It wouldn't do me any good if he says yes . . . (*That the wish for a baby occurs as a nightmare points up the conflict between the wish and the overwhelming anxiety in respect to having further burdens. She likes to take care of infants. "When they are small like that, they are no problems." She has six already and doesn't think she "should be so greedy." Until her infants begin to walk, they are no burden to her and remain totally under her control. She remarks that the youngest of her children "is starting to get out on her own and she is feeling her oats." She thinks that "maybe I will have one out of six that I will conquer." As she vacillates between admitting and denying the trouble she is asking for, I confront her.*)

Dr.: You have to be honest with yourself. You are eager to have another baby as your little one is beginning to grow up and be a little bit more independent. Your husband is saying no, but you know ways of getting him to—

Pt.: Not right now. I have too much ahead of me. I have to go and have my teeth out, so it seems it's one thing after another for at least a few months, so I better not.

Dr.: Your little one is a year old. With your other children have you wanted another baby after a year?

THE CASE OF THE CONQUERED WOMAN

Pt.: The minute they start walking then I say they are not a baby anymore.

Dr.: The minute they start walking.

Pt.: Once they are a year old they don't want to be rocked because that means sleep. They resent all that. We both like to be able to pick them up and love them, but they only want that when they seem to be infants . . .

Dr.: Well, let's say, then, that this dream of yours was simply saying in your sleep, in a disguised way, that you want another baby.

Pt.: Could be. If it's meant to be, it will be.

Dr.: What do you mean, if it's meant to be?

Pt.: Well, even if we follow rhythm. If you're meant to get pregnant, you get pregnant.

Dr.: Especially if you want to be.

Pt.: So I am just waiting to see, that's all. If I don't have any, then I will just have to be satisfied with the six I have, which isn't too bad.

Dr.: Not at all. I think I know a man who doesn't know it, but he's going to have another child.

Pt.: I don't know about the man knowing it. But the in-laws, I don't know if they will like it or not.

Dr.: His side?

Pt.: No, not his side. His side doesn't have anything to say.

Dr.: You mean your mother?

Pt.: It's my side that has to help me out. I am terrible when I am pregnant. I need all kinds of help, and I am in bed for three months when I start.

Dr.: So you mean it's your sisters.

Pt.: Yes, they have to.

Dr.: Not your mother?

Pt.: God, no, she can't help me now.

Dr.: They will all have to help you, and if they knew you were pregnant or want to be pregnant, they will raise hell.

Pt.: They will leave the country. Maybe by now, after six, they will just say, "Go ahead and go take care of yourself."

Dr.: They won't help you?

Pt.: I don't think they can. One is worn out from taking care of my mother, and the other one lives a ways. She's the one who has had the hardest life, but she is always there whenever I need her. She figures you are supposed to have them, and you're supposed to have them one right after the other.

Dr.: The thing that I question is that I know you want very much to have another baby, or at least try to have one, and that you can talk your husband into it.

Pt.: I don't know what the dream meant, but I know that I conquered that feeling and I went back to sleep. That's what used to bother me, so I didn't question it any more when I got up this morning. I was glad that I had gone back to sleep and didn't dream any more.

Dr.: At least you know that you want another baby, and that it's on your mind.

Pt.: Not all the time.

Dr.: How often do you have relations with your husband?

Pt.: Well, like I say, the one night after my period and seven nights before.

Dr.: Twice.

Pt.: What do you mean twice?

Dr.: How long do you have relations with your husband?
Pt.: Seven nights before.
Dr.: Each night?
Pt.: Mmmm.
Dr.: So you have enough sex?
Pt.: I think so. I don't know about my husband, but I do.
Dr.: Seven nights before.
Pt.: And one night after.
Dr.: Will that be eight times then?
Pt.: Sometimes. Sometimes maybe only two or three times.
Dr.: But as much as eight times in the month?
Pt.: Yeah. I don't take chances. Not unless I want another one.
Dr.: Who keeps track?
Pt.: I do.
Dr.: Whether it's safe or not safe. Have you ever—
Pt.: I don't try to lie because he is going to go out and check the calendar, so I
don't dare lie. I have the calendar marked, anyway, so he can look at it and
tell. A couple of times I have said it's the right time, and he said no because
he had checked the calendar. That was a good six months ago, and she
wasn't very old then.
Dr.: Did you know that you had made a mistake?
Pt.: Yeah, but I didn't want to do anything wrong. I didn't want to practice
birth control.
Dr.: Have you or your husband practiced any other method than rhythm?
Pt.: No.
Dr.: All right. So you want a baby. Now what else has been going on? (*She is
active about the house in ways that she had not been for years. She continues to go out alone and notices rising tension when she enters a store to
do her shopping. She forces herself to continue and is aware that the
anxiety disappears if she does. This leads her to talk about her fear of
closed places. Her reactions are typically phobic. In church or in the
movies, she must sit where she can make a rapid exit; she is afraid that she
will become sick and faint. Eleven years ago she passed out once at work;
although she never has since, she has remained fearful about doing so.*)
Pt.: If I faint, I may not wake up. I am afraid of dying.
Dr.: The fear that you will die.
Pt.: I used to fear that if I fainted I wouldn't come out of it, and I didn't want
to pass out on the bus, and I didn't want to have the children with me.
Dr.: And this has been going on for how long?
Pt.: Eleven years.
Dr.: Never before?
Pt.: No.
Dr.: Eleven years beginning—do you remember when it began?
Pt.: When my daughter was a year old, Jessica.
Dr.: Do you remember where you were?
Pt.: It was at the movies.
Dr.: What was it that you were seeing?
Pt.: A movie about head surgery, brain surgery.
Dr.: And you had to get out.
Pt.: I didn't get out, I just left my seat and went and got a drink of water and

came back and sat there. I was with somebody, and I didn't want to make them leave.

Dr.: Jessica was a year old. Tammy is four years younger than Jessica. Do you remember how come you waited so long between Jessica and Tammy?

Pt.: Because I was so sick. I would say at least three years I was bad, and I was on all kinds of tranquilizers and all kinds of pills.

Dr.: You were bad?

Pt.: I had been to a few doctors. So I didn't have any children, and then I started feeling a little better.

Dr.: Do you remember when you wanted another child?

Pt.: Not really. I would say maybe a year before I had Tammy. I started feeling a little better. I think that's when I went on the Doriden.

Dr.: What were all these pills given to you for?

Pt.: They were tranquilizers. Every doctor I went to, they claimed it was just nerves.

Dr.: What was?

Pt.: The reactions, the heavy palpitations and the perspiring, and I couldn't sleep nights. And they tried one pill after another.

Dr.: Were you having any particular difficulty with Jessica?

Pt.: No, no. She was a good baby. She wasn't sick or anything, or hard to handle. No, it just happened. Like I say, I had taken a bad attack of arthritis, and the doctors thought it was rheumatic fever because I couldn't walk and use my arms. As fast as that left, I had the other attack in the movies.

Dr.: Who were you with?

Pt.: In the movies? One of my neighbors.

Dr.: Is she still a neighbor?

Pt.: Oh, yes. She sat with me for four years. Actually, she used to come in and stay with me. I used to be afraid of being alone, and I never went out. I was so bad I couldn't even go out to the front steps. I went to my obstetrician, and he told me that everything was backfiring—all the tranquilizers.

Dr.: What is this neighbor friend of yours like?

Pt.: She is a happy-go-lucky person. I don't see too much of her now because her children are all grown up and she's working.

Dr.: Older than you?

Pt.: I would say about five years older.

Dr.: Were you quite attached to her?

Pt.: I wasn't attached to her, but she was one of these persons you could depend on if you needed somebody in a hurry—in an emergency.

Dr.: Did she tell you what to do?

Pt.: No, she's not that kind of person. She wouldn't tell you what to do. She would just sit and talk, and you didn't do anything while she was there.

Dr.: Did you come to depend on her a good deal?

Pt.: I think I had to call her only two or three times for emergencies. I had to go out—when my father died and a couple of other times.

Dr.: I will see you next Friday.

Pt.: And I hope I won't be late next Friday.

The patient has arrived a bit late and is breathless, both from hurry-

ing and from fear that she would lose the whole time as a kind of punishment for not being precisely on time. Her need to be good pervades all her activities, the important as well as the unimportant. She is looking well and feeling "good." Of special interest is the appearance of a nightmare the preceding night. It is important from at least two points of view: (1) She was able to manage the episode without calling on her husband for help and was able to return to sleep; (2) the nightmare comes at this moment in the treatment and occurs the night before this interview. In such instances, it is reasonable to believe that a major stimulus for the nightmare was the knowledge that on the next day she would be coming for her interview. The nightmare rather blatantly conveys her conflicted wishes about having another baby. She is a woman who likes babies only while she is able to exercise t 'al control over them. On the other hand, it is during pregnancy that she is able to satisfy quite fully her own dependent needs. She gets her family to take practically full-time care of her. Thus, the wish to have a baby at this time may be seen to arise not only as a repetition of a similar wish coming five times after the irth of her first child, but also as a way of becoming acceptably sick, relieved of all responsibilities, and of gaining a childlike attachment at the time when the treatment interviews are drawing to an end. Her ambivalence about good health and its attendant responsibilities, versus illness and dependent attachment along with their secondary gains, may be understood as reflective of the early failure to separate herself from her mother and to achieve a sense of reasonable individuation and an adult identity. Why this did not happen has been well illuminated in the details of her relationship with her mother. In the treatment situation, she is up against the same early issue as time begins to run out. Active consideration of termination must begin in the next interview.

Tenth Interview

Pt.: I'm feeling good, very good.

Dr.: You are good?

Pt.: Mmmm. Except I am a little warm from sitting out there (*in the waiting room*).

Dr.: A little too warm?

Pt.: It was hot coming over on the bus, too, but it was nice outside. I have been pretty good this week. I went to school.

Dr.: You went to school by yourself?

Pt.: Wednesday night, yeah.

Dr.: How did you do?

Pt.: Good. Haven't been there since last October.

Dr.: Last October?

Pt.: Yes, just before my mother went into the hospital. Not since. So I went back Wednesday. Which was good. It felt good to get out. And I went to the dentist. Felt good all week.

Dr.: Feeling good. Sleeping?

Pt.: No. Not on account of myself. The other two little ones came down with the chicken pox, so I haven't slept too much. I sleep in between—when they sleep.

Dr.: Always something.

Pt.: As long as it isn't me, I don't mind. As long as I am not nervous, I can stay up and it doesn't bother me.

Dr.: Don't you get a little fed up with it sometimes?

Pt.: No.

Dr.: You get over one thing—and another—

Pt.: And another.

Dr.: And then something else.

Pt.: I figure this is it now, for a while, I hope. Then the colds will start again.

Dr.: Oh, so you really don't feel it is the—

Pt.: I hope it's the end. Now I have to start thinking about myself and the dentist.

Dr.: What about that?

Pt.: I had two taken out, and I have to go back and have five out. I am not looking forward to it, but if they have to come out they have to come out. Once that's done I hope things will be different. At least I won't have any teeth ache. That will be one thing I'll be rid of.

Dr.: So you have taken care of your teeth, and you are feeling good.

Pt.: Feeling good.

Dr.: Doing things.

Pt.: Like I say, I went to school, and I have been baking up a storm.

Dr.: Have you really?

Pt.: Which isn't good for anybody.

Dr.: Why not?

Pt.: None of us need it. Actually, we are all overweight. But it's something different, something to do, and I have been letting the children help me, which I haven't done that for a long time—you know, letting them putter around flour and everything.

Dr.: Well, you certainly have been doing very good.

Pt.: I feel I am. Then I am going shopping today by myself.

Dr.: Maybe I missed it. You are letting the children putter around the flour, something that you—

Pt.: Haven't done that for a long time—since the oldest ones were little. I never had the patience.

Dr.: To let them mess up a little bit?

Pt.: Oh, yeah. They have fun doing that.

Dr.: I am sure they do. Were you ever allowed to do that?

Pt.: Oh, yes, I could always cook at home.

Dr.: That was one thing you could do.

Pt.: Yes, which I always liked to do. Maybe that's why I like to let the children do it now. But when I was—I couldn't be bothered letting them. You know, they were always in my way.

Dr.: Sure.

Pt.: Pushing them away—which I am not doing now.

Dr.: So you feel happier about it, too.

Pt.: Yes, the oldest ones, too. The oldest are remarking about it—how the little ones are getting away with murder, getting to do things which they don't remember they used to do. All they remember was when I was always yelling and complaining.

Dr.: Well, you have a good report today.

Pt.: I feel good, too, accomplishing all this.

Dr.: You should. Should I give you an A report card?

Pt.: I think I deserve it this week. And I am not going home. I am going shopping.

Dr.: Double A . . . You should be very pleased with yourself.

Pt.: I am. I realized that Wednesday night when I made up my mind that I was going out to the school. Although I didn't go alone. I took my daughter because she goes to school, too.

Dr.: She takes the—

Pt.: No, they have a different course for the children. I took her along because I didn't want to carry everything myself. I had too much to carry.

Dr.: Was it that, or were you afraid?

Pt.: No, no. I couldn't carry it on my own.

Dr.: You weren't kidding yourself?

Pt.: No, I was just determined, because I had called my niece to see if she would go and she said no, so I still went—which ordinarily I wouldn't have done before unless I had a ride. But this way I walked and discovered I am overweight because I was huffing and puffing. So I think a diet will help, too.

Dr.: You remember it wasn't too long ago you weren't able to eat a darn thing.

Pt.: It seems to go from one extreme to another—couldn't eat before and now I can't stop. I don't know whether getting false teeth is going to be good or bad. I will be able to eat all the sweet things that I haven't been able to eat for years.

Dr.: A real challenge for your will power.

Pt.: I think I have been doing good. I just hope it keeps lasting like this.

Dr.: You hope what?

Pt.: It lasts.

Dr.: Why should it not?

Pt.: I don't know. I think that it will. When I look back, I think it was about a month ago I was ready to give up. But now I have been able to fight a lot of things off.

Dr.: What do you mean you thought you were ready to give up?

Pt.: One day—I forget—it must have been a month ago when I came in and I said I hadn't felt good and I felt that I was halfway over before that.

Dr.: Yes.

Pt.: And when I came in, I said it was all going down the drain.

Dr.: You felt that half the battle was won.

Pt.: Was won.

Dr.: What was the other half? Do you remember?

Pt.: Coming here.

Dr.: Yes. You do remember.

Pt.: I remember it now.

Dr.: Coming here was the other half. How about that?

Pt.: Well, it wasn't as bad as I thought it was because I found out that as the weeks progressed that I was doing better and, more or less, looked forward to coming now. Like I said to my husband, I don't know what I am going to do with Fridays when I am all through. I can't keep asking him to keep coming home on Fridays to let me go out. (*Avoiding separation from me.*)

Dr.: When did you tell your husband that—you didn't know what you were going to do with Fridays?

Pt.: Last week. This has gotten to be a habit now. I am going out on Fridays, and I don't always go right home. He can't keep taking off from work, either.

Dr.: It's going to have to come to an end, isn't it?

Pt.: Fridays will have to, I know that. I mean, like after I'm through.

Dr.: When is that?

Pt.: Well, whenever you say I am through, which I figure two more weeks—will be twelve weeks.

Dr.: Two more weeks after this will be twelve weeks, you are right. That will be on February seventh. Are you thinking any more about that?

Pt.: You mean?

Dr.: Just two more weeks.

Pt.: Two more weeks.

Dr.: After this.

Pt.: Not so much having two more weeks. I have been thinking more or less what I have accomplished in the other weeks. I think that I have accomplished a lot.

Dr.: I think that you have, too. No question about it. You were also saying, as you said to your husband, you don't know what you are going to do now.

Pt.: I will miss getting out on Fridays.

Dr.: Let me get it straight. What do you mean, you will miss getting out on Fridays?

Pt.: I never took a day off during the week, you know. Like he said, when I don't have to come here, just take Saturdays.

Dr.: Instead.

Pt.: And go off.

Dr.: I see. So you will miss the Fridays for that reason.

Pt.: Well, it really isn't—don't know how to put it—entertainment. But it's out. It seems as though no matter where I—it's still just out, away from the house.

Dr.: Do you think that you will miss me? (*Termination, separation from me must be pursued.*)

Pt.: I will miss talking. I don't ordinarily talk at home to everybody. I don't confide in them. Well, my husband I do. But I feel like I empty my basket with little things that's bothering me.

Dr.: So it's not that you will miss me, but rather that I am someone to talk to.

Pt.: I have enjoyed your company.

Dr.: You have enjoyed that, too.

Pt.: I like to meet people.

Dr.: I am just trying to, you know, keep you honest.

Pt.: Mmmm.

Dr.: It isn't simply a matter of having somebody to talk to, but after all, I am also somebody.

Pt.: Oh, yes.

Dr.: Yes, and you have enjoyed my company.

Pt.: Mmmm. I feel that I don't have to please you anymore, like I did in the beginning.

Dr.: You certainly did feel that you had to please me. You don't feel that way now?

Pt.: No. I don't feel that I have to please anybody. Maybe my husband and that's all. Now I find that I can sit on the phone and say, "I am sorry, but I can't make it." "I can't go here," or "I can't go there."

Dr.: And you are not going to say to me anything that you think I want you to say.

Pt.: No. There was something that I was going to say, and I can't think of it. It couldn't have been too important.

Dr.: Maybe it was very important.

Pt.: If it was that important, I wouldn't forget so fast. Mmmm. Well, what will I do when the twelve weeks have gone by? I mean, do you think that I am going to need any more? (*She pursues another tack to avoid the end. It is also the kind of question that tends to shake the confidence of the therapist and lead him to make inappropriate assuring remarks.*)

Dr.: What do you think?

Pt.: Well, I don't think so. I mean I haven't only learned to get over these feelings that I had, like the dizzy spells, nor pay attention to the pains—I have learned to accept a lot of things which with your help we have pointed out different things—when I got home I would think them over and see how foolish it was that I let them bother me, you know.

Dr.: But you are—you do wonder whether you will stay this way when we're through.

Pt.: I do and I don't. I think it's more or less up to myself whether I stay this way, and as long as I, you know, stand on a firm foot and don't let people bother me, which I am doing now. Because I know I am supposed to do certain things, should do certain things, but I push them aside and do whatever I want.

Dr.: You are able to manage things if you want.

Pt.: If I want to, yeah. So I think that I have accomplished a lot.

Dr.: I do, too.

Pt.: But—why couldn't I have seen this myself?

Dr.: It's not easy to look at yourself.

Pt.: There are a lot of things that you brought up, my husband brought up. But why I didn't pay any attention to him? That's what I don't understand. Like he used to say, "Don't let this one bother you; tell him to go to blazes," and it used to bother me.

Dr.: Did I tell you to do that?

Pt.: In a roundabout way you brought out of me that it was bothering me and I shouldn't let it bother me.

Dr.: Did I say it shouldn't bother you?

Pt.: No . . . (*Once more, I go into detail with her as to whether she had made changes for the better out of her need to comply with what she felt were my wishes. I do not accept her immediate replies as final so that she may have ample opportunity to examine her motives as carefully as possible.*

THE CASE OF THE CONQUERED WOMAN

She comes out finally in a direct, genuine manner and says, "I am not doing it to please you. I am doing it to please myself or to help myself. These are things that have accumulated over the years, and I know that they are there. When you ask me questions, you break them out into the open, and I thought about them twice instead of shoving them back into my mind and trying to forget them.")

Dr.: You said a little while ago that you don't have much time left.

Pt.: No. In the beginning it seemed like an eternity—twelve weeks. And here ten weeks have gone by, and I think I am so much better than I was when I first came. Two weeks left. Maybe I am going to accomplish a lot more in just the two weeks. (*"In the beginning, it seemed like an eternity": How directly and beautifully this woman, natively intuitive, expresses child time, time that would stretch out interminably in expectation of never-ending warmth, comfort, and sustenance.*)

Dr.: Let's go back to that time when you mentioned, where you said half the battle was won, and now you have to fight the other half, which is—

Pt.: Coming here.

Dr.: What does coming here really mean. Does it mean coming here to this place?

Pt.: Coming for help. Coming for help and helping myself.

Dr.: The other half. Half the battle is won, the other half is coming here. What is the "here"?

Pt.: Help. I don't know how to put it. The other half is I have to come for help, and when I don't have to come—

Dr.: Here—but to whom?

Pt.: To you, I imagine. I am not seeing anybody else in here.

Dr.: You imagine?

Pt.: I am not seeing anybody else here. I am not coming to anybody else for help.

Dr.: So that when you say half the battle is won, the other half is coming here. And coming here is—

Pt.: Coming for help from you. And then I figure—

Dr.: Here—is coming to see me.

Pt.: And when I am through with that, I am going to help myself, which I haven't been able to do since—eleven years now. I think that's why it's more or less at the back of my mind all the time.

Dr.: But since you said half the battle was won and the other half is coming to see me, then you must have also felt that that was something of a battle for you—to see me.

Pt.: Well, more or less. It was coming every week and bringing everything out and reliving a lot of things, which seemed like a chore in the beginning and then the middle there—it doesn't seem to bother me so much now. But there was a time there when I was coming, and then I was talking about my mother and different things like that—and it was really bothering me, and I would go home and I would think about that, and then I would get over that part. So I am—I figure—(*She struggles to avoid the confrontation with the therapist as a significant figure.*)

Dr.: So now you figure yes, there isn't much time left, and you are going to try to do still more in the few meetings that we have.

Pt.: Well, mmmmm . . .

Dr.: Have you had any other thoughts about the fact that we only have two more meetings after today?

Pt.: I often wonder if you think that I am doing as well as I think I'm doing. Do you think I need any other help? I mean, like I say to my husband, I don't know whether it will be all over, or I am going to need any more help someplace.

Dr.: What is your preference?

Pt.: Well, today I can say that I feel I don't think that I will need any more. I always have the feeling I might go into it in the future, but I will just have to wait until I come to it instead of worrying about it. I'll just wait and see. It's a bad habit always worrying about what is coming.

Dr.: You are always looking for some disaster.

Pt.: No, not a disaster now. Just wondering. Like you say, I'm wondering am I going to be all right or am I going to be—

Dr.: No, I didn't say it, you said it.

Pt.: When I mentioned two more weeks.

Dr.: Yes, and you wondered whether you will be all right.

Pt.: Be all right, yeah. That's something that I just can't seem to correct—that part.

Dr.: Do you have any idea at all what might make you wonder whether next week or the week after that you might feel as well or better, rather than the other way?

Pt.: No. I don't know why I do it. Like my husband says, "Live for today; forget tomorrow. Let it come as it will." I am always planning ahead. Like even today, I started to plan a vacation already instead of waiting. (*For the first time in ten years, she is planning on a short vacation with her husband and without any of the children. While this is obviously a progressive move, coming at this time in the midst of my exploration about the end of time, it must be seen as being an avoidance device as well.*)

Dr.: Do you have any feelings about the idea of finishing here and not coming here any more?

Pt.: None other than I have mentioned. Once I am through with this I will tackle others, and there will be different things I want to do concerning my health.

Dr.: Like what?

Pt.: I want to have my teeth taken care of, and my eyes. So I figure if I finish this—take care of my nerves—

Dr.: What do you mean when you say *if* you finish this?

Pt.: Did I say it?

Dr.: Yes.

Pt.: I meant to say when I finish.

Dr.: Well, you know when you are going to finish it.

Pt.: In two weeks. So I figure if I can take care of that, then I wanted to have my eyes taken care of. I didn't know if my nerves had anything to do with that, so I figured I would take care of my eyes after . . . (*Another attempt to avoid the issue of separation. She tries to steer me away from it by injecting one additional constructive plan after another. All of these aim at telling me that she is well and is planning ahead. Anything but to examine closely the separation that must take place.*)

Dr.: Have you had any nightmares?

Pt.: No, not since the last time, thank goodness.

Dr.: Do you remember what we talked about in connection with the last nightmare?

Pt.: You felt it was because I wanted another baby that I dreamt that—which I had a hard time trying to—

Dr.: You already knew what you said—that you do want another baby . . . (*She continues the question of having another baby especially since all her plans will lead her toward becoming "a new woman." In fact, she is full of ideas about keeping busy, including the possibility of getting a job, although she has not worked since her marriage. There is a sense of overactivity about her, and we may understand this as a further adaptive effort. That is, the activity serves to conceal depression from herself; depression as a result of impending separation.*) Anything else that you have been doing more so than usual?

Pt.: More so than usual. Staying off the telephone. I ignore the telephone—don't make any calls.

Dr.: Calls to—

Pt.: Today when I was coming here I remembered that I hadn't called my mother, and then I started to think I hadn't really called anybody all week. I used to get out of bed, feed the children and send them to school, then I'd sit right down and call my mother every morning. And then I would call my sister. But I haven't bothered calling anybody. I call my mother once a day but not at a specific time, which I was in the habit of doing. It was routine, and if she doesn't hear from me she wants to know what happened. I just tell her I was too busy.

Dr.: So you did call her today.

Pt.: No.

Dr.: When did you last call her?

Pt.: I called her yesterday, but I didn't talk long.

Dr.: So that's different, too. You are not calling anybody in your family to—

Pt.: And like I am going out tomorrow, but I know she feels I am going down there. But I'm not going.

Dr.: Who feels it?

Pt.: My mother.

Dr.: Thinks you are—

Pt.: She asked me if I was coming, going out Saturday, and I said yes. I said I don't get the opportunity to go out myself, so see you maybe Sunday.

Dr.: What did she say?

Pt.: Nothing. She said, "Well, no, you don't get out." I said I don't—I said I only go to doctors and hospitals and dentists. I said I am not going over—

Dr.: When she said, "Are you going out Saturday," does that mean—

Pt.: She thought maybe I would say, "Well, no, I'll be down," which I didn't.

Dr.: And she didn't fuss.

Pt.: No. And I told my sister, and she says to me, "Did you say you would be going down?" I said, "No I'm going out."

Dr.: Did your sister say anything?

Pt.: "Good."

Dr.: She said, "Good for you?"

Pt.: So, I'll go out.

Dr.: You went into the lion's den and nothing happened.

Pt.: No. I think she's come to the point that if she wants somebody to come down, she's going to have to change a little bit and take us when we can get there. I have enough to do. I go if I'm rested and take care of her and do her work for her. But if I'm not rested, I've got my own to do first, and she's so alone she certainly can't be as messed up as I can be.

Dr.: And she's all alone.

Pt.: She manages. (*Now we see that she is effecting a very satisfactory separation from her mother. To her surprise and gratification, she finds that she can alter her pattern of response to her mother and gain a respectful, non-retaliative return.*)

Dr.: All right. Let's see, we have two more meetings. I'll see you next week.

Everything is "good," and she is doing very well in every way. She has resumed her ceramic classes, is going out alone, and is apparently embarking upon a full rehabilitation program for herself—to fix her teeth, eyes, get a part-time job, and "be a new woman." She no longer calls her mother every day nor at a precise time of the day. She is taking no medication of any kind, and, despite the continuing impression one gets that she wishes very much to please me, it does seem that she is experiencing and enjoying a new sense of freedom and independence for the first time. She indicates awareness of impending termination when she remarks, "I'm going to miss having Fridays off." We then discuss the fact of there being only two more meetings left, whereupon she promptly wonders if she will remain well. Since I offer her nothing to suggest that there will be anything more after the next two meetings, she then answers her question affirmatively for herself. It is interesting to note that she had once before planned to get a job and was pregnant when she applied. Will she do this again, to ward off the fear of being independent?

Eleventh Interview

The patient came in today wearing a new dress and, for the first time, uttered not a word for about five minutes.

Dr.: I'm sorry, I'm late.

Pt.: It's not what you would call late.

Dr.: Why not? Five or six minutes late.

Pt.: You are forgiven. I went over to the clinic to make an appointment to have my eyes examined. I found I was a little nervous today.

Dr.: You were a little bit nervous? What from?

Pt.: I more or less got up that way this morning. I don't know what to relate it to.

Dr.: You didn't feel this way yesterday?

Pt.: No, no. I have been doing good.

Dr.: Till this morning.

Pt.: This morning. And I've noticed—like around—I think that I mentioned it before—around period time, if I don't have the pressure in my head, then I feel anxious instead.

Dr.: How close are you to your period?

Pt.: A week. And yesterday I was very warm. My head was hot, and then that went away and I was fine. This morning I got up and I was debating whether I felt good enough to come or not.

Dr.: Really? You mean you felt that bad?

Pt.: Edgy.

Dr.: Edgy?

Pt.: Yeah, so I took a cab and came anyway instead of missing my appointment.

Dr.: You said you debated with yourself as to whether you should come?

Pt.: If I felt good enough—

Dr.: And how did the debate go?

Pt.: I figured it was better to come while I felt that way, maybe—you know.

Dr.: The other choice would have been to do what?

Pt.: To stay home. But then again if you have a toothache, you don't wait till the toothache goes away before you go to see the dentist. That's how I felt.

Dr.: At the dentist? Dentists generally hurt people, don't they, in the process of helping?

Pt.: It may help. There is a little pain there, but that's the same with most things.

Dr.: Do you think there will be some pain here?

Pt.: No. Like I said, if I came I would know whether I was putting—how will I put it—light on the matter, you know.

Dr.: As to why—

Pt.: Nervous and edgy.

Dr.: It happened this morning.

Pt.: Yeah. And nothing seemed to bother me to get me that way.

Dr.: What was the thing that was different about this morning from yesterday, the day before, and the day before that?

Pt.: When I got up I felt a little nauseated and then a little light-headed.

Dr.: Today. What was different about today as compared to yesterday?

Pt.: I felt good the other day.

Dr.: Anything different about today?

Pt.: You mean when I woke up?

Dr.: Like the day that is facing you.

Pt.: Nothing.

Dr.: Nothing different when you awakened this morning so far as the day is concerned?

Pt.: No, not that I can think of.

Dr.: I know something.

Pt.: Coming here.

Dr.: Well, of course.

Pt.: I don't think that bothered me. I didn't think about it when I woke up. All I thought of was that I felt sick.

Dr.: I am sure you didn't.

Pt.: But then when—well, I will stay home, and then, maybe I better go even though I don't feel good.

Dr.: But you will say and agree with me that one thing about waking up this morning that was different from other mornings—

Pt.: That I was coming here. I don't know if that bothered me or not, subconsciously.

Dr.: And then you found yourself wondering if you should come or whether you should stay home.

Pt.: Not whether I should come, but whether I felt good enough to come over. I figured if I took a cab I would get here faster than taking a bus. Once I came and had a little commotion down at the desk, down at the cashier's, and that kind of took my mind off something, whatever was bothering me.

Dr.: You mean that when you got here—since you arrived here you have been feeling better?

Pt.: Yeah. Because I was so confused.

Dr.: How do you mean?

Pt.: I went down to pay for my appointment, and I gave her extra money, and the girl got it all mixed up, and from one thing to another I was getting confused, and I wasn't thinking about myself.

Dr.: So when did you begin to feel better?

Pt.: When I came upstairs. I noticed that I wasn't so edgy.

Dr.: When you came upstairs?

Pt.: Then as I was sitting there waiting I started to get nervous just sitting there. I have to keep going.

Dr.: In other words, you have mixed feelings about seeing me today.

Pt.: No, no, no. It was sitting there alone. I like to keep busy doing something. I don't sit down ordinarily.

Dr.: You mean you don't like it. But why should sitting there alone start to make you nervous again? What were you doing there?

Pt.: I was having a cigarette.

Dr.: Yes, but what were you waiting for?

Pt.: Waiting for you to come.

Dr.: You were waiting for me.

Pt.: And then I didn't know if I had been late running around, that was all. And then I started to feel, you know, a little light-headed again, and then you came along and I was all right . . . (*She has begun to react rather acutely to the impending separation. She experiences confusion in managing details of her entry to the clinic, although she is entirely familiar with the procedure. Then I "came along and I was all right." She regains her defensive balance and begins to deny that anything unusual could account for her nervousness. I continue to press her in respect to the relationship of the onset of her anxiety and her visit today. She blurts out, "I know that I went to sleep thinking about it last night." She does not understand why her visit today should have troubled her because she had actually been looking forward to it all week. She had even remarked to her husband about her visit to me out of her preoccupation with a particular aspect of the treatment: "How the time has gone by, you know. All these weeks have already passed and everything. It seemed like an eternity when it first started.")*

Dr.: How many times do we have?

Pt.: Left? One.

Dr.: How do you feel about that?

Pt.: I don't know. I was thinking about that yesterday. To me it feels as if I was going to school.

Dr.: Oh, you were thinking about it yesterday?

Pt.: Yesterday. Thursday night when I was going to school. I went to ceramics, and I was thinking of coming here Friday, and I said, "Gee, that's just like going to school when you are going to graduate but—that—it doesn't bother me."

Dr.: But graduations sometimes are kind of a bothering period in life. What does graduation mean to you?

Pt.: Like when you are all through school—college—and you have achieved so much schooling. Not that I have achieved something.

Dr.: What else does graduation mean?

Pt.: That's all I can think of.

Dr.: You finish school and achieve a certain amount or kind of education, and what follows?

Pt.: Oh, you have to work when you graduate from school. You have to go out and get a job and work out what you've learned and take over yourself.

Dr.: Go on your own.

Pt.: Mmmm. And I try to figure things out.

Dr.: Do you have any qualms about that—after next week you will be on your own?

Pt.: Just be more or less wondering how things will be, but I just have to wait to find out.

Dr.: But you do have these wonderings.

Pt.: I have to have that, I think.

Dr.: You say you would have to have that. I am not going to flunk you in this course.

Pt.: Well, I couldn't really sit here and say, "Oh, I am going to be fine after next week."

Dr.: I want you to say exactly what you feel.

Pt.: I found out a lot of things about myself, and now I feel I can handle them probably myself.

Dr.: But you have your qualms.

Pt.: Yeah. I am still wondering if I will still be able to handle it the way I can handle it now.

Dr.: Next week you will get your diploma. You will graduate this school. You will be on your own, and that's okay by you, but you sometimes wonder whether—

Pt.: I will be able to make it. I'll make it. I know that I am not going to feel that much better just because I am not coming back but—

Dr.: Wait. Tell me that again.

Pt.: I mean coming every week. I feel I come every week, and I am getting help—help—and it helps me out till the following week. So I am not going to be all better, as if I had a cold and the next week it's going to be gone, because I am all through coming. What is bothering me will still be there—just have to work it out myself—that's how I feel right now.

Dr.: Do you think that you will miss coming here?

Pt.: Probably if I get a spell or something. I will be looking forward to help, but I will have to do that myself.

Dr.: You think that only if you get a spell or something that you will think about and wish you were coming here.

Pt.: If I feel I need—

Dr.: You said you feel good. Do you think you will miss seeing me?

Pt.: No. I don't think that I will miss coming here. Like I said last week.

Dr.: I didn't say coming here.

Pt.: I like your company and everything, but I don't think I will miss you that way.

Dr.: Are you telling me the cold honest truth?

Pt.: I don't know how to put it.

Dr.: Just put it very simply, honestly.

Pt.: No. I just as soon not have to come. If I don't feel well, I am not going to sit there and say, "I wish I could go to see Dr. Mann." Instead I will probably put on my coat and go out. I hope that's how I feel, anyway.

Dr.: That's very good.

Pt.: That's how I am looking forward to feeling.

Dr.: I can tell the way you were smiling that you like seeing me.

Pt.: Like I said to my husband—he asked how I was making out and every-thing—what seems important to me, everybody in the family will think it is so minor that it shouldn't be bothering me, but you would listen to me. I told him that's what I liked about coming. Things that seem important to me seem important to you.

Dr.: Yes.

Pt.: Where they don't mean anything to anybody else.

Dr.: So you think to yourself. If you feel well, of course, that's what you want. But regardless, you don't think that you will miss coming, seeing me—are you sure?

Pt.: I don't know whether I am saying the right thing or not.

Dr.: You have to say whatever is in your own mind and is truthful. It has nothing to do with my feelings.

Pt.: Like I said before, I will miss your company, but I won't miss sitting here and discussing myself. It's like you meet an acquaintance, friends, and you like to be with them.

Dr.: Yes.

Pt.: But you wouldn't want to have to think of them, "Well, I have to go see that person now because I need help." I mean, if I would see them in the street, I would be pleased and happy to see them. That's how I feel. I hope I haven't hurt your feelings saying that.

Dr.: Now what was there that you just said that you think would hurt my feelings?

Pt.: Well, that I won't miss you.

Dr.: Some people do and some don't. You are privileged to feel whatever it is that you feel.

Pt.: Well, I appreciated everything. Like you have helped me. I don't think I could have done it myself, that's for sure, because I have been this way for years and I haven't gotten anywhere.

Dr.: But you are afraid that it would hurt my feelings if you say that you will not miss me.

Pt.: Mmmm, professionally. I'll put it that way.

Dr.: That you are not going to miss me professionally. Does that mean that you will miss me personally?

Pt.: Personally, as an acquaintance.

Dr.: But not professionally. You just as soon have had enough of talking about your problems. That makes perfectly good sense that I can understand—

Pt.: I have to fish for words sometimes. I used to find it easy to say things but I get kind of befuddled with the right words.

Dr.: So next week is graduation.

Pt.: Oh, I hope so.

Dr.: Of course, it's going to be. Do you have any doubts about it?

Pt.: A lot of things could happen in a week.

Dr.: What can happen in a week?

Pt.: Many things. It will be graduation if—

Dr.: If—

Pt.: If everything is all right when I get here. I hope I live to see it. Like I feel— it's that I have accomplished a lot.

Dr.: But do you have any thoughts in your mind that you will live to next week to get here?

Pt.: You never know. It used to bother me at one time, but not now. That's another thing I have learned to look at with a different point of view.

Dr.: So that if you are around next Friday, and there are no serious accidents, and we're not in an atomic war—

Pt.: Oh, please.

Dr.: Or anything like that, you will be here . . . (*She then tells that she made a deal with her husband that he would be willing to babysit two or three nights a week after he has graduated so that she could work. Her oldest daughter works three nights a week, and she would not consider hiring any teenager to come in as a babysitter. She says that going to work a few nights each week would be like an entertainment for her, a means of getting out of the house and doing something other than visiting someone.*) . . . Well, you are talking like a graduate, aren't you?

Pt.: I don't know.

Dr.: Job, get your eyes fixed up, teeth fixed, and go out into the world.

Pt.: And fight it. That's about the only way I can see it. If you can't fight it, you might as well put yourself in a room and stay there. That's what I've been doing for too long. So I figured if I fight it, I can get out and enjoy myself . . .

Dr.: Your aim is to get out, graduate and move out into the world the way graduates are supposed to.

Pt.: Before I am too old, and then I will find myself in a room soon enough.

Dr.: How many graduations have you gone through?

Pt.: Just school, grammar school and high school.

Dr.: Do you remember how you felt?

Pt.: Mmmm. I felt elated, I felt good.

Dr.: I am sure. Any other feelings at the time?

Pt.: I can't remember. I imagine I felt proud of myself, but I can't remember back that far. It's a long way back . . . (*Note the pride in accomplishment. In good measure, the confidence of the therapist in his ability to be of help in so short a course of treatment is related directly to the increase in self-esteem which all persons experience when, with a little bit of help, they can go on to do still more for themselves. Her association to termination as a graduation is to the point.*)

Dr.: Last week you told me that you once before had had plans like this about getting a job and something happened.

Pt.: I got pregnant with my last baby. Or I was pregnant at the time and didn't know it.

Dr.: So that took care of that idea about working.

Pt.: I couldn't work that summer. I was too sick, but I didn't forget about it. I kept saying as soon as the chance comes up I'll try it . . . (*She speaks of some intention to go to work outside the home and then, interestingly, promptly reveals once more her conflict between establishing herself as independent or as dependent. Much earlier in her married life, intentions to go out to work were effectively thwarted by her becoming pregnant. She begins now to talk about the two possibilities, getting a job or getting pregnant. She disclaims all responsibility for the latter, "If I get pregnant, I just have the baby and take care of the baby. There isn't much you can do about it. I figure if I have a baby, then that's God's work. If it's in the cards, it's meant to be. If I'm going to have them, I'll have them."*)

Dr.: That's exactly the point. I think this is one way that you can keep yourself at home.

Pt.: Maybe subconsciously I don't want to work, I don't know, but I would like to get out. I would like the baby, and then I would like to go out, too. I would like to work, too, but I can't do both.

Dr.: No, because you know from earlier experience that when you get pregnant, you know what happens.

Pt.: What happens to me?

Dr.: Yes.

Pt.: I get sick.

Dr.: And what does that mean?

Pt.: That means I stay put for about three months, and I can't do anything.

Dr.: Who takes care of you?

Pt.: I take care of myself and my husband helps. Between the two of us we manage. But sometimes I get bad, and I have to have somebody come in to help me do it. The last one wasn't too bad, but that's because I had the older one helping me. I didn't have to ask anybody to come in.

Dr.: Now that you and I are almost through here—one more meeting—you have plans for yourself. You are going to have an eye checkup, you are getting your teeth taken care of, and you think that maybe in the spring, after your husband is through, you would like a job. At present you are also still going to ceramics class. All these things are getting you out. Next week you will graduate from here, and you might be tempted to stay in.

Pt.: In the house, you mean?

Dr.: Yes, and how could you do that? Well, one way you could stay in the house is to get pregnant.

Pt.: I don't stay in the house that much when I am pregnant.

Dr.: You do get sick.

Pt.: If I am sick, I'm in, but if I'm not sick, then I am out. But—oh, no, I don't want to go back to staying in the house. You mean, the way I was before? No, I would really have to be sick to think of that.

Dr.: You know, when you came to see me, we talked about your being dis-contented, irritated—with what?

Pt.: With the house and children.

Dr.: Yes, with all the burdens on you, and you felt like a slave.

Pt.: Mmmm, that's how I felt.

Dr.: You had to do whatever your mother said or anything that your sisters said. The only person that you could control was your husband. You were someone who felt terribly controlled, afraid to go out, and had to just stay put.

Pt.: That's how I was, but I think now that I have gotten out I have been fighting this. I don't think that I want to go back to it.

Dr.: Yes, I know that you won't want to go back to it, and I am saying that one of the things you had better watch out for is you may get yourself preg-nant and get yourself back in the house.

Pt.: I have been thinking of that, too, and I was wondering if I would feel any different now being pregnant than before.

Dr.: I don't know.

Pt.: Because I was nervous and taking all kinds of pills before. The doctor thought that caused a lot of my trouble with my pregnancy, the pills I was taking. So I want to learn how I would be, which probably isn't a good idea either. So, the only way I would know is if I got pregnant.

Dr.: Well, that's something you could arrange.

Pt.: Yeah. Right now I guess it's a little too much—too much going right now. As much as I want another one, I think I better wait a while.

Dr.: Don't do it for me.

Pt.: No, there are too many things going. I want to see my husband finish school, and I think that that would be a little more of a burden on his shoulders—even more so than my own . . . (*We shift now to a consideration of her more immediate feelings. She has been sleeping much better but has had one episode of palpitation in the night that frightened her. She hears that rapid beating of her heart as she lies on the pillow and gets out of bed in fear. Her fear is that she will hear her heart stop, that she will die. She regains her composure when she hears her heart rate slow down.*) The fear of death doesn't bother me half as much as it used to.

Dr.: Everybody has some fear of death. This whole thing about palpitations, you are afraid your heart is going to stop and you are waiting to hear. It slows down and you feel at ease again. I think it was last week or the week before that we talked about your fear of passing out—where you would faint, but you would know it, too.

Pt.: I would know it.

Dr.: I think that your difficulty in falling asleep is related to that, too—to know what happens when you go to sleep.

Pt.: Well, it could be the chance that you are just not going to wake up.

Dr.: You might get up in the morning and find yourself dead.

Pt.: That would be something—to get up and find yourself dead!

Dr.: Seriously, I think that this might be one of the things that interferes with your sleep. You are afraid to go to sleep because you might die. (*An exceedingly significant disclosure as to the source of her insomnia.*)

Pt.: And yet I want to sleep . . .

Dr.: Were you always afraid of death?

Pt.: No.

Dr.: When did it start?

Pt.: It never really bothered me much until my father died.

Dr.: Ever since—ever since his death it has kind of bugged you. Tell me about your father's death.

Pt.: He had a heart attack, and he didn't die right away. Then about four days later he was rushed to the hospital, and we were waiting for the doctor to examine him but he was dead and we didn't know it. They came out and told us he was dead. All I can remember of his illness was the way he used to rub his chest all the time with the pain. And this friend of ours, this priest, he was always rubbing his chest; he had a pain. After that, every time I had a pain in my chest I thought I was going to die. I must have felt bad. I didn't go to the hospital where both of them had died. Every time somebody mentioned that hospital, I said, "If you go there you are not going to come out alive." That stayed with me for quite a while. I remember one time I had a—I forget what you call it—something under the ribs, a cold, and I thought I was having a heart attack, and my husband rushed me over to that hospital. But it wasn't a heart attack. All I have to do is have a pain in my chest and I feel kind of—but now I just say I have a pain, and I just keep going. I know the other night I had an awful pain, and I said, "Maybe you are going to die"—

Dr.: Who did you love more, your mother or your father?

Pt.: I think I was closer to my father. He was the type of person we could always go to with something that was bothering us.

Dr.: He was a nice guy.

Pt.: Mmmm, I liked him.

Dr.: Maybe you even loved him.

Pt.: I loved him. He had his faults but I felt his good points overthrew his bad points. Of course, everybody has one or two bad points, but I was close to him.

Dr.: Still miss him?

Pt.: Yeah. I miss him a funny way. I go looking for him when certain things happen. Like if something will come up in the house and it needs to be repaired, I will just head for the telephone and forget that it's six years—

Dr.: You still find yourself going to call him?

Pt.: Going to call him, yes. And yet I never had to do anything for him. So I do miss him; we all do.

Dr.: I don't know about the rest of your family, but you—

Pt.: He made a deep impression on me. I don't know if that's half of my sickness, too. (*We have seen how much the dynamic process of treatment revolved about the controlling relationship she suffered with her mother reflected in the nature of the transference to the therapist. Now as termination nears, the transference shifts from the therapist as mother to the therapist as father. The loss of father is soon to be repeated within the treatment.*)

Dr.: How do you mean?

Pt.: Well, the way I am afraid of heart attacks, where I was always thinking about him every time I had a pain. I used to wonder, but I found out that I can have the pains and I am still not dead.

Dr.: You can go to sleep without dying, and you can get here next week and still be alive.

Pt.: Oh, I hope so. I hope I am going to be alive more than one more week. I would like to live a little bit longer. I think that after these eleven years I have something to make up.

Dr.: But you still miss your father and think about him when something comes up in the house, and you almost go to the phone.

Pt.: There isn't a day that goes by when I don't think of him . . .

Dr.: Is there anything when you think about your father? Is there anything in a particular way that you think about over and over?

Pt.: No. When he would come to the house and he would argue with the children—whenever the children, the little ones, were doing something wrong, that's when I mostly think of him. I think, "If your grandfather was here you wouldn't do that," and that's when I think about him. Because we used to laugh when he used to start yelling at the children, and he would be yelling at them and the next breath he would be going out to buy them candy or something. So that's how I think about him every day, because I have the children always doing something wrong to bring it into my mind, and when there is something to be done I will say to my husband, "Well, if my father was living, it would be done" . . .

Dr.: Well, was he somebody you could talk to?

Pt.: Oh, yes. We could go to him with just about any kind of problem and he would listen to us. My mother wouldn't have the patience. If it was something that my husband and I had an argument over, I could go to my father but not to my mother. She would turn around and say, "I told you not to marry him."

Dr.: Your father would listen.

Pt.: And he would tell us what he thought whether we liked it or not. If he thought we were wrong, one of us, he would tell us.

Dr.: Do you miss him in other ways, besides when something has to be done and you remember that if he were around he would do it?

Pt.: We used to go out with him.

Dr.: Who is we?

Pt.: My husband and I. We used to all like to get together and go out.

Dr.: Go out with him?

Pt.: We would have parties. We haven't had any since he's gone.

Dr.: Have you thought of him particularly—your father—this week?

Pt.: This week—no more than usual.

Dr.: Does that mean every day?

Pt.: Yeah, but I mean—just a quick thought if something turned up. I haven't' dwelled on it. There was a time when I used to just sit and think and think.

Dr.: When did that stop?

Pt.: I think that only lasted about a year or so.

Dr.: After he died.

Pt.: Mmmm. It's hard to believe because he was never a sickly man and he seemed—and went so fast.

Dr.: How old was he?

Pt.: Seventy, but he seemed like a person who was just never going to die, you know. He was indestructible, and he could do anything—come close to death and nothing would happen. I mean that wasn't just my opinion; that was everyone that knew him felt that way. And he never bothered you. He had a very happy outlook on things, and it doesn't seem that none of us have his outlook. I guess we all more or less take after my mother, which I wish I had taken after him. It would be nice to have the outlook he had.

Dr.: He was very important to you, and you have been missing him every day for six years.

Pt.: He used to be all I needed when I was sick.

Dr.: Would you like to see him?

Pt.: Would I like to see him? Well, my time will come. I will see him when I get there. I am not going any sooner. I am not in that much of a hurry.

Dr.: You're not in a hurry?

Pt.: He will keep wherever he is. He can wait for me better than me going to meet him.

Dr.: I think so, too.

Pt.: I will see him when the time comes, and he must be happy where he is. He hasn't come back.

Dr.: He hasn't come back?

Pt.: He must be pretty good. When they go, they don't come back.

Dr.: Do you know anybody who does come back?

Pt.: No. Well, it can't be too bad, I suppose.

Dr.: But you miss him, nevertheless.

Pt.: Oh, yes.

Dr.: We will have our final meeting next Friday.

The patient is preoccupied with the rapidity of the passage of time—it had seemed so long, and now we are almost through. Her reference to graduation is a way of expressing adolescent concerns about independence, career, marriage, and so forth. It refers also to the more infantile anxiety in respect to separation from the nurturing, sun-giving mother. She has found a way of maintaining her own need for dependence and avoiding one kind of adult responsibility by becoming pregnant. This may seem to be a strange assessment of what is and what is not a responsibility. For her, however, the rewards that lie in being able to call upon others to take care of her and in attaching an infant to her even as she was attached to her mother, to whom she has been ambivalently attached through all her growing and adult years, compensate to a considerable extent for the drudgery of everyday burdens of caring for a lot of children. Attempts to open her direct feelings about me meet with partial success only. She will miss my "company"; perhaps this is as much as a religious, somewhat prudish woman can allow when her feelings about me and about leaving me are being explored. We then learn more of her close relationship with her father and the extent to which he continues to exist for her each day. Her continuing impulse to phone him whenever some need arises in the house during the day suggests what she might wish to do after her treatment is over.

Twelfth Interview

Pt.: I feel like I have been here all day.

Dr.: What time did you get here?

Pt.: I got here about 12:30 . . .

Dr.: Tell me about you. How are you?

Pt.: Not too good today.

Dr.: Yes?

Pt.: Or yesterday or the day before. I get nauseated. I think it's my teeth.

Dr.: Why should your teeth—

Pt.: I have an awful taste in my mouth. It comes from a tooth that is open to drain.

Dr.: Could you vomit?

Pt.: I did.

Dr.: Appetite?

Pt.: Very poor.

Dr.: Nervous?

Pt.: No, not actually nervous—aggravated.

Dr.: Are you?

Pt.: I am more inclined to say that, rather than nervous, because I feel good otherwise.

Dr.: Aggravated on account of what?

Pt.: Being nauseated constantly, and I don't like to go out feeling that way.

Dr.: When did it start?

Pt.: I would say around Tuesday or Wednesday. It wasn't too bad, but then Wednesday night and Thursday and today I have been more or less unbearable.

Dr.: Has it just started to drain that way?

Pt.: No. It's been draining about three weeks, but I figure that now it must have gotten the best of me. And then I have a cold on top of it.

Dr.: Then it has been draining all this time?

Pt.: Yeah.

Dr.: This is nothing new then.

Pt.: No.

Dr.: What is new is that something is getting you down.

Pt.: Well, it isn't—I have had that but it hasn't stopped my appetite before.

Dr.: As of Tuesday.

Pt.: Monday or Tuesday. I noticed I wasn't eating too much.

Dr.: Do you think it has anything to do with the fact that you are going to be through with me today?

Pt.: No, I don't think so.

Dr.: Nothing at all?

Pt.: I haven't even given that a thought. I was aggravated with the other—just wishing that was all over.

Dr.: Haven't even thought about this.

Pt.:   I have been too preoccupied with my teeth. I went to school Wednesday night and I had a candy bar, which I haven't had for months. It ended up my bottom teeth started to ache, so then I started to get discouraged. I don't know what I am going to have to face.

Dr.:   I can tell you what you are going to face.

Pt.:   You mean with my teeth or myself?

Dr.:   You, yourself.

Pt.:   I don't know.

Dr.:   Do you know what you are going to have to face?

Pt.:   Have to face getting my teeth out; that's going to bother me. I don't know what else you have in your mind.

Dr.:   That's all you are thinking about now, about your face.

Pt.:   Right now that's all I am thinking of, because they really have been bothering me.

Dr.:   Do they hurt now?

Pt.:   I can't eat. If I start eating, they ache, and when they start aching, I get irritable. I think it has come to the point where they have to come out. I have to go tomorrow, so maybe they will tell me something.

Dr.:   Going to the dentist tomorrow?

Pt.:   I was supposed to be going for an impression, but I don't think I will.

Dr.:   Have any nightmares?

Pt.:   No, I have been sleeping pretty good.

Dr.:   I am sure that helps.

Pt.:   I have noticed that I go from eleven or twelve to seven in the morning now, which I haven't done in a long time.

Dr.:   The main thing, then, is your teeth are bothering you, and there is also irritability.

Pt.:   I don't like the way I feel.

Dr.:   You mean—

Pt.:   Nauseated.

Dr.:   That's not a pleasant feeling.

Pt.:   You feel like you are pregnant constantly.

Dr.:   I will ask you again, are you?

Pt.:   No, I am not. I wouldn't mind. I would rather be pregnant and know where it's coming from, instead of just being sick all the time.

Dr.:   You remember that you were nauseated and without appetite once before.

Pt.:   When I had been taking the pills, and I stopped taking them, and—

Dr.:   And once before, more recent than that.

Pt.:   I think that was when my mother was in the hospital.

Dr.:   It was right after you started—

Pt.:   Around November.

Dr.:   Right after you started here with me. Do you remember you lost—

Pt.:   I had lost nine pounds.

Dr.:   And you weren't eating and felt nauseated all day. Is it anything like that?

Pt.:   No.

Dr.:   How is it different?

Pt.:   I felt nauseated before, but now I vomit.

Dr.:   How often?

Pt.:   Two or three times yesterday and twice this morning, which is unusual and gets everybody in the family guessing, and the children are looking. They

Dr.: are all guessing and looking in vain. They remember when I am pregnant I have morning sickness. So this morning they are all looking at their father.

Dr.: Really?

Pt.: But he reassured them I just didn't feel good. Otherwise I feel pretty good.

Dr.: Do you know what I think? I think that you are sick to your stomach and nauseated and vomiting because this keeps your mind off something else.

Pt.: What?

Dr.: The fact that after today you are not going to see me.

Pt.: It might be, but it's kind of a foolish thing.

Dr.: No, it's not a foolish thing to be doing. It's not that you are making yourself sick. For some people it's very difficult, harder to face up to missing somebody. They would rather suffer sick stomachs or aching feet or whatever than an aching heart.

Pt.: Well, no. But it's an awful way to, to—it's not the predicament to put yourself in.

Dr.: You don't do it because you prefer it that way. You can be afraid of missing somebody. Have you ever missed somebody?

Pt.: Only my father.

Dr.: Did it hurt?

Pt.: No.

Dr.: It didn't hurt?

Pt.: Well, hurt—how? I didn't have pain or anything.

Dr.: What kinds of pain are there?

Pt.: Pain that I would feel. I didn't have any pain.

Dr.: No?

Pt.: Mentally I think that I suffered, because I was thinking constantly. That's the only way I could put it.

Dr.: Mental pain can be pretty painful, can't it?

Pt.: It can, because you don't seem to think or do anything else but that one thing. (*The power of her defenses is apparent. Eagerly, she comes to the appointment forty-five minutes early. She has prepared herself for this last session with a host of somatic symptoms, which clearly serve a diversionary purpose. A certain degree of concrete thinking is also summoned in defense. Thus, when I ask her if missing her father hurt, she can only think of it in terms of having or not having chest pain. All this only reinforces the necessity for me to remain fixed to the goal of dealing with the patient's feelings about termination in direct terms, since there is no time left to explore the symptoms at any length. Moreover, sufficient data about the symptoms have been amassed already as to provide clear understanding of what is transpiring.*)

Dr.: Does it sound completely strange, or unlikely, or even possible that you would miss me?

Pt.: I don't know. You mean, coming here and getting help from you?

Dr.: Miss me. You have come to know me by now. What am I saying that seems so strange to you—that you might miss me.

Pt.: I don't know. I know I have been looking forward to being on my own again. I have in the back of my mind, and I am going to make it.

Dr.: But no feeling of missing seeing me.

Pt.: No, I don't think so.

Dr.: Does it sound strange to you as I say it to you now?

Pt.: No, no. Maybe in a couple of weeks from now I could answer that better, but right now I am anxious to see if I can handle myself. Can I get around without coming and talking to you. That's what I am anxious to find out.

Dr.: Let me put it this way, what kind of questions do you raise in your mind when you say to yourself that you are anxious about how things will be?

Pt.: During the week when things bother me, I always say to myself, "Well, I will take care of that Friday when I go to the doctor." Now I will have to say, "Well, I will just have to settle it now by myself." The past few weeks I have always stored up things. I would be coming, and I would be able to talk to you. But now I will have—waiting to find out if I am going to be able to do that by myself.

Dr.: Now you know that you will not be able to store everything up and wait until Friday to see me. How do you feel about that?

Pt.: A little nervous. I am not really sure of myself on that—more or less hoping that I will be able to handle it. But there is that little idea in the back of my mind, "What if I can't?" That's what I am waiting to find out.

Dr.: What do you say to yourself in answer to the question, "What if I can't?"

Pt.: I haven't been able to answer that.

Dr.: You haven't gone any further?

Pt.: No, I figure I am going to have to be off before I can answer that. I will have to find out when something arises to see what happens. It will be a challenge to myself. So I keep hoping that if something comes up, I will be able—I feel if I can handle something once, I should be all right—give me courage to, you know, go on. It's not going to be easy, because it's been too easy storing things up and waiting until Friday to come here.

Dr.: It's been too easy?

Pt.: Anything that has come up I say, "Well, I will let that go until Friday," instead of really, well—some things I have taken, but anything that really bothered me, I just set it aside.

Dr.: Save it for Friday.

Pt.: For Friday.

Dr.: And after today, there's no more Fridays. Do you have any feelings about that?

Pt.: Just a little nervous. It's a feeling like I were going on a new job or something and to know if I am going to be able to handle it or not . . .

Dr.: The thing that makes you nervous is that up until now, something would come up and you could say to yourself, "Well, okay, I will wait until Friday." But this is the last Friday. Now you won't be able to say, "I will save it for Friday," so that you can't turn to me. Is that what you mean?

Pt.: Yeah.

Dr.: Nobody to turn to then.

Pt.: Well, I have my husband to turn to.

Dr.: How did that work out before?

Pt.: A lot of answers I got from him were similar to what I got from you, but I just didn't pay any attention to him. There were a lot of things he advised me to do.

Dr.: What did I advise you to do?

Pt.: Not advise. I mean if I came to him with a problem, he would listen to me.

Dr.: And he would offer advice to you?

Pt.: Not a solution, but he would give me a roundabout answer, but I wouldn't accept it.

Dr.: Was there anyone else you ever listened to when you would present a problem?

Pt.: The only one I ever listened to was my mother.

Dr.: You did everything she—

Pt.: Whichever way she gave me an answer I did that, whether it was the right solution or not.

Dr.: You did it.

Pt.: But like I say, I can turn to my husband. I think right now I shouldn't have to. I should try not to turn to anybody and try to solve my own problems.

Dr.: You told me last week that there used to be somebody you could turn to.

Pt.: Oh, my father.

Dr.: Did you listen to him?

Pt.: Oh, yes.

Dr.: Was it different from listening to your mother?

Pt.: Yeah, because my father's opinions wouldn't necessarily be in my own favor all the time. If I gave my mother the same problem, she would always make it my husband's fault.

Dr.: Did you respect your father's opinion, but not your husband's?

Pt.: If I didn't feel good, or nervous or something, I just figured that my husband didn't have the medical knowledge or whatever.

Dr.: Neither did your father.

Pt.: I never confronted him with my health. It was like problems with the house. Until I came here, I was just looking for somebody to side in with me, and my husband didn't. He would tell me what he thought was best for me, and if I didn't well . . .

Dr.: Last week you told me that there are times when you think of your father quite often. And there are times when you actually think of picking up the phone to call him about something, and then you remember, of course, that he is dead. You know, this means to me that not only was your father so very important to you, but that you—in your mind, it is as though he is still alive. (*She has given sufficient evidence to warrant this direct confrontation and interpretation of her preconscious, if not unconscious, fantasy about her father. He is known to be dead but continues to be felt as alive. In this way she is able to keep him with her. The result, of course, is that she has never achieved separation from her father, and we know of her attachment to her mother. Her next response speaks directly to this.*)

Pt.: That's possible. But I can't keep thinking of him that way.

Dr.: Well, if you go to the phone to call him—

Pt.: I think it's just such a strong feeling I had for him and I just can't let him go.

Dr.: Yes, exactly. People that we have strong feelings for we don't like to let go.

Pt.: And yet, if he were living and suffering, I could let him go.

Dr.: But he isn't living.

Pt.: Only the memories. That's the way I think of it now.

Dr.: So much so that, as you said, you could start to the phone.

Pt.: If something happens.

Dr.: And then remembering that of course, you can't call him.

Pt.: Yet there are other people that I think of, but not so strong.

Dr.: I am sure.

Pt.: And yet I was attached to them.

Dr.: Yes, but obviously your father—

Pt.: With my father I look—I feel deep down if he were here, I would have half the responsibility that I have with my mother. I think that's why I feel the way I feel. I am constantly thinking of him.

Dr.: I think also that aside from the sinful fact that you love him—or does that not sound right?

Pt.: Oh, no. I loved him, but now that you bring it out I don't know why I should be so possessive in thinking like that.

Dr.: How do you mean, possessive?

Pt.: That I should let him go and not be thinking about him. I don't know. Now that we have talked about it, I feel maybe I am wrong.

Dr.: Wrong? Do you think that I am saying that you are wrong?

Pt.: That it isn't right to be thinking of somebody—

Dr.: Why not?

Pt.: No, that's why I am asking you.

Dr.: Are you going to do what I say?

Pt.: No, no. I was just wondering if there was something wrong with me thinking often like that. If you told me to stop it, I couldn't stop it, naturally.

Dr.: It's not a question of is there anything wrong. As you put it yourself so very well, maybe you can't let him go, and we do that with people that we very often need.

Pt.: But I don't think that is hurting me.

Dr.: Who says it is hurting you?

Pt.: Well, I thought that's the impression you were under.

Dr.: That it's hurting you?

Pt.: Mmmm.

Dr.: How did you get that idea?

Pt.: It bothered me the way you were talking about it.

Dr.: What I was trying to say to you was that by holding on to him in that way, then you don't have to miss him.

Pt.: I don't miss him that much.

Dr.: And by not missing him as much, you have saved yourself some pain.

Pt.: Well, possibly.

Dr.: After all, if you think of calling even though you know that you can't, then it doesn't hurt as much.

Pt.: Oh, it does when you realize that you can't talk to him. But then, after so many years—then you say, "Well, that's kind of foolish to think of picking up the phone," and you remember—

Dr.: Maybe it's foolish, but certainly you feel it. We got around to this by this question that you have been raising to yourself, "How are you going to make out after we are through here?" You are saying that you could talk to your husband, and yet you remember talking to him, but somehow you didn't respect what he had to say. It didn't carry the same weight somehow.

Pt.: It's probably an awful thing to say, but now that I have come here and spoke to you, and many things that you have said, he has already said—so I feel now that maybe he knows a little more than I know, and I should give him the benefit of the doubt. Of course, when he did speak to me and tell me anything, it would be things that he had done. Like, he used to say, "Why get nervous because you can't sleep?" and that used to bother me because he would say he didn't sleep, but yet he didn't get nervous over it.

Dr.: And what did I tell you?

Pt.: Well, you didn't tell me that you couldn't sleep nights. You just brought out—I forget now what you brought out about my not sleeping. I know we talked about it a couple of weeks ago—because I am afraid if I go to sleep I may not wake up. But see, my husband would always say he tried this, or he tried that, and it worked. And I always say what works for one doesn't work for the other, but I would never give it a fair try. Now maybe I might listen to him and see how that works out, because he hasn't always been wrong.

Dr.: No, I am sure not. So that's one possibility, for you to speak with your husband. Anything else you might do?

Pt.: In regard to what?

Dr.: If you feel that you are nervous about something, wondering about something.

Pt.: There is nothing else I can do except what I have been doing and try to overcome it and face it and just push it aside and try to do something. And that's what I have been doing. I had several spells, and I just got dressed and went out and tried to get over it.

Dr.: And you did.

Pt.: Mmmm. But I still find that I am a little nervous if I have to go out, but I still go. If I conquered that much I ought to be able to conquer the rest eventually.

Dr.: That's true.

Pt.: But today where I didn't feel good and I was coming, my husband said, "You are not going to be through. You are going to go through twelve more weeks." And I said, "No, I am not," and he said, "Yes, you are." He was pulling my leg because I didn't feel good. In other words, that I shouldn't think about it, just get busy and forget it. He thinks I dwell on it too long.

Dr.: Why would he say that?

Pt.: Just to tease me. So we ended up back and forth, and I forgot it for a while. And then he always turns around and says, "You are not as sick as you thought you are." And then I get mad. But I *was* sick.

Dr.: He says you are not as sick as you thought you were?

Pt.: I was just sitting there, and he kept saying, "Well, don't sit there and think about it. Get up and do something." And I kept saying, "I don't feel good enough." And he said, "Eventually you are going to have to get up and get ready and go to the hospital." Then he said, "Maybe you will have to keep going if you don't get out of this—get over this," and I said, "Oh, no." He was fooling, teasing me back and forth.

Dr.: Has that thought been in your mind at all?

Pt.: About what?

Dr.: That you might have to go for twelve more times.

Pt.: No, I never thought of it because—well, I feel I am coming here, but nobody is forcing me, and if it was suggested I would have my own choice to make, I imagine.

Dr.: If what were suggested?

Pt.: That I would have to come for any more treatment.

Dr.: No, I am not going to suggest that.

Pt.: Yeah, but I mean, I think that I would have a free choice in the matter, so it's not bothering me. I never gave it a thought until today when my husband started.

Dr.: Can you say anything about how you are feeling now?

Pt.: Right now?

Dr.: Yes. Do you know what you are feeling now?

Pt.: Well, I feel fairly good, but I don't know what you mean.

Dr.: What feeling are you presently having?

Pt.: I feel free; my mind feels free.

Dr.: Right now. Anything else?

Pt.: Right now I don't feel sick.

Dr.: Of course not.

Pt.: That's not fair though.

Dr.: What do you mean fair?

Pt.: That when I leave here, then I am going to feel sick again.

Dr.: You don't have to.

Pt.: I suppose just because I have been talking, I can talk myself right out of it.

Dr.: No. You haven't talked yourself out of it. You are with me, and while you are with me you are not missing me.

Pt.: A feeling of security?

Dr.: You are not missing me now, but when you leave you are going to miss me. But you are not the kind of girl who allows herself to miss people.

Pt.: Oh, I do.

Dr.: I don't think so.

Pt.: Like I miss my children if they are not around.

Dr.: Oh, sure, but I mean people. It's understandable that as a mother you might miss your children if they are gone.

Pt.: Do you mean acquaintances?

Dr.: No, I mean people who become or are important to you in a very kind of personal way.

Pt.: The only person that I have ever missed other than my immediate family was the priest that we were acquainted with, and when he died I made a statement I would never get attached to anybody again.

Dr.: Did you really? When was that?

Pt.: That was two months before my father died.

Dr.: Never get attached to anyone else again. I think that you are attached to me whether you know it or not.

Pt.: Well, I might have a feeling of security. It's—like if I got to the hospital when I have my children.

Dr.: I think it's more than a feeling of security. I think that you like me.

Pt.: Maybe.

Dr.: You mean you don't know?

Pt.: Well, I like you, yes. I mean, I have enjoyed your company. But like I said before, I am glad that I won't—

Dr.:	I know all about that. All I am saying is—
Pt.:	I don't want—
Dr.:	Can you admit to yourself that you like me?
Pt.:	Mmmmm.
Dr.:	You can say?
Pt.:	I wouldn't have come back the second time if I disliked you.
Dr.:	Never mind all that. I am only asking you one simple little thing. Can you admit to yourself that you like me?
Pt.:	Yeah, all right.
Dr.:	Now you are not saying that—
Pt.:	No. I don't see why you should have to ask, because I wouldn't come back if I didn't like you.
Dr.:	I don't care about that. I am asking you something else. All I am asking is whether you can admit to yourself that you like me—no ifs, ands, or buts.
Pt.:	I do like you.
Dr.:	Is that your own honest answer?
Pt.:	Yes.
Dr.:	That you like me. If you like me, then you are going to miss me.
Pt.:	I know that I am going to find myself, you know, I don't know for how long, but in the course of the day wishing I could come to talk to you if something arises. I know I am going to face that.
Dr.:	And I am suggesting that you are going to face or have to face something else—that it is not only that you like to talk to me but that you would like to talk to someone that you like.
Pt.:	Mmmmm.
Dr.:	Which happens to be the same person.
Pt.:	Yeah.
Dr.:	And therefore you are going to miss me.
Pt.:	When you put it that way—I mean, before when you just asked me am I going to miss you, I didn't know.
Dr.:	You can't admit those things. It's very hard for you to because you are afraid of pain, like you said. I don't mean physical pain.
Pt.:	Mmmm. Mental pain.
Dr.:	Mental pain. As much as missing somebody like you said about the priest. He meant a lot to you, didn't he?
Pt.:	Oh, yes. That's why I said I didn't like how I felt after he was gone.
Dr.:	You can turn on or off, whichever way you like.
Pt.:	That's true, but in this case it isn't as if you are—
Dr.:	Say it.
Pt.:	As if you had died. Where I used to go to this priest if anything bothered me—I could talk to him. Whether I could ever call and make an appointment to see you if I needed to come, I don't know. It's a different feeling. It isn't a lost feeling.
Dr.:	It isn't—
Pt.:	It isn't a lost feeling that I would have for this priest friend of ours.
Dr.:	No, not yet, because you are still here. But you may get this feeling.
Pt.:	That I have to talk to—
Dr.:	Yes. Not that you have to as much as you would like to.
Pt.:	That I would like to. Yes. I will just have to handle it with myself, that's all.

Dr.: That's true. On the other hand, what I am trying to help you with now is to let you know that you are a human being. You and I have talked about a lot of things here, and I know that you like me. If I am wrong, you say so.

Pt.: No.

Dr.: That's no sin. It's all right for people to like—

Pt.: Oh, I know that.

Dr.: And I know that you are going to miss me, but you will try to keep that out of your mind. You're that kind of gal.

Pt.: Probably, I don't know.

Dr.: You protect yourself from certain painful things. I am not criticizing you, I am just telling you the ways that you have to protect yourself . . .

Pt.: Because I think that years ago I probably got attached to everybody.

Dr.: Might well be.

Pt.: I know that I was attached to the people that I worked with. When I left work I felt bad. Even when I went to the hospital to have the children, I would get attached with who might be in the room with me.

Dr.: And you were attached to your father.

Pt.: Mmmm.

Dr.: And he left you.

Pt.: And that's it.

Dr.: And you have become attached to me. And if you make believe it isn't so it doesn't change it. I am saying that you have become attached to me, and then suddenly—gone.

Pt.: It's hard to face.

Dr.: Like your father.

Pt.: It seems that everything that I do—not everything that I do—but it's a sudden break, most things that happen to me.

Dr.: Like—

Pt.: Like meeting people, and I can enjoy the company, and then all of a sudden they are gone. I know that there are people that have friends and they go on for years and years.

Dr.: Well, that's friends.

Pt.: But mine either move or they die.

Dr.: That's true. But your father was more important; your mother, too.

Pt.: I still have her here.

Dr.: Right. Priests are important, too. What do you call a priest?

Pt.: What do you mean, if I am friendly with him? Father.

Dr.: Father.

Pt.: Well, that's always the way I have been taught to address them.

Dr.: Well, of course. What does father mean?

Pt.: For a priest, it's a type of respect.

Dr.: What else does it mean?

Pt.: And then there is father, your own father.

Dr.: Yes. You see you are thinking about your father and so often are ready to call him. That tells us how much you were attached to him, how much you wish he was around to talk to him or tell him, "Look, please come over and help me with this, or help me with that." The fact that he is dead and that you think of calling him only makes it even stronger how much you wish he were around. Now I am saying that we are going to be finished in just a few minutes, and you will go on your way. I am saying that you should know that you are going to miss me. This is human—just like you miss your father—and you are going to wish that you could call me.

Pt.: Call you?

Dr.: But you won't be able to.

Pt.: No, I know.

Dr.: Because I am dead.

Pt.: You are not dead. You are alive. You are here.

Dr.: Yes, of course, but just the way it was or is with your father, you have the same feeling.

Pt.: Same feeling. That's right.

Dr.: And I think it's important for you to know that you have such feelings, and that you do want to be on your own.

Pt.: Oh, yes.

Dr.: But you would also have the feeling that the only way you can be on your own is not to let yourself be attached.

Pt.: To somebody.

Dr.: To me.

Pt.: But yet I know I am going to think of you as I am going on.

Dr.: To think of me?

Pt.: Yes.

Dr.: You are right. And what will you think of me. What is it going to feel like?

Pt.: I don't know. I imagine I will be wishing I could just call you and tell you what is bothering me, but I know that won't be possible.

Dr.: Just like your father. You might also at some times feel angry with me.

Pt.: I don't know why.

Dr.: Why not?

Pt.: You haven't done anything to make me angry.

Dr.: Perhaps.

Pt.: I have come, and I have spoken to you, but I think I have helped myself a lot, too.

Dr.: That's true.

Pt.: So I don't think that there is anything that I could blame you for.

Dr.: Except one thing.

Pt.: Possibly being friendly, being attached.

Dr.: No, I think probably because you know that I am not dead.

Pt.: So I would be angry for that?

Dr.: Not for that. But if I am not dead, then what follows?

Pt.: I don't know.

Dr.: I am around, aren't I?

Pt.: Yeah.

Dr.: And yet you can't call.

Pt.: Well, that would be just like having medicine and knowing that I shouldn't take it.

Dr.: Knowing that you can't, that you are not allowed to take it. You won't like that sometimes.

Pt.: I will have to get over it. I mean, I have been in this predicament before.

Dr.: What I am saying is that I think it's important for you to know your honest feelings, that there may be times when you will feel angry with me for not being further available to you.

Pt.: I can see that.

Dr.: There I am just a telephone away.

Pt.: That's right and I can't—

Dr.: I don't think you are going to like that sometimes.

Pt.: Probably not. If something really—

Dr.: If you are honest with yourself, then you will recognize this and it might help you. And there will be times when you won't be angry with me or with somebody else, but you will want to see me because you will miss me, and it's important to be honest with yourself about that.

Pt.: That makes sense.

Dr.: But you are not a stick of wood, you know.

Pt.: Oh, no, I hope not.

Dr.: You have feelings.

Pt.: I have feelings, but sometimes they work in the wrong way.

Dr.: You are right.

Pt.: And that's what a lot of my problem is.

Dr.: When you say they work in the wrong way, what do you mean?

Pt.: I don't know. I think that I fight it a lot.

Dr.: In which way?

Pt.: Offhand, I don't know.

Dr.: Well, I will give you an example. How did you feel before you came in here today?

Pt.: I felt sick.

Dr.: That's one way you fight your feelings.

Pt.: But, like I said, I don't think—I knew it wasn't bothering me coming here today.

Dr.: I *know* that it was bothering you.

Pt.: All week all I have been thinking of was the dentist, and I don't want to go there.

Dr: I know that you were thinking of the dentist so that you wouldn't have to think about coming here for the last time.

Pt.: I could be, but I know all I had in mind was the dentist.

Dr.: This is your way of fighting off certain feelings. All you could think of was the dentist, feeling sick to your stomach, nauseated, and vomiting. But no thought about the fact that this was your last visit here with someone where you feel that you have gotten some help and with someone you like—no thought about that.

Pt.: So I used the dentist.

Dr.: This is one of the ways you avoid your own honest feelings. Next time when you feel nauseated or have a headache—not every time—but especially if you come down with some other symptoms, ask yourself—

Pt.: Why.

Dr.: What it is that you are feeling about somebody else or something else that you are not allowing yourself to feel—instead you are feeling this.

Pt.: Getting sick.

Dr.: Yes, getting sick. What it is that you don't like.

Pt.: So instead of fainting sometimes I invent a sickness.

Dr.: Don't be hard on yourself. You know, it's not that you are a bad person to invent sicknesses, you simply find it hard to face what you feel about people.

Pt.: Mmmmm.

Dr.: Do you follow me? There **may be** times when you will feel irritable and angry and not know quite why. And you will have to ask yourself who are you angry at; or you might find yourself feeling quite sad, and you ask yourself who is it that you are sad about.

Pt.: Why couldn't I have thought of that? Like if it is brought out, it seems so simple and yet I couldn't see it. It was there and I couldn't see it.

Dr.: You are human. This is the way people are. We all try to avoid pain.

Pt.: Mmmm.

Dr.: Mental pain.

Pt.: That's a funny way of doing it, though.

Dr.: Yes, but it's a very human way. If everybody knew that by themselves—

Pt.: I could see your point there.

Dr.: I wouldn't have any work to do.

Pt.: You wouldn't have a job.

Dr.: That's right. All right, you have your chance now for one question before we quit.

Pt.: Only thing I can think of—anything that *really* bothers me and I can't face it, then what will I do?

Dr.: I think that you can face it and will be able to.

Pt.: I am glad that you have that much faith in me. Like, I'll probably have that much faith in myself eventually, too. That's the only question I can think of.

Dr.: Thank you, very much.

Pt.: Thank you, Doctor.

In view of the stout resistance put up by the patient in this final interview, one could easily visualize a further series of interviews aimed at her defenses concealing affect. However, the final interview should be understood and managed solely in respect to the accumulated data and to the sequence of unconscious dynamic events that have been activated by the treatment process. The power of the unconscious insistence to continue earlier ambivalent attachments is instantly recognized in the fact of her becoming symptomatic during the twenty-four hours preceding this final appointment. Nausea, vomiting, poor appetite, and a constant sense of being pregnant speak eloquently to powerful oral fantasies in both their acquisitive and rejecting aspects, hence ambivalent. She makes a number of attempts to continue the treatment, first through her husband's remarks, and then directly herself. At the very end of the interview, she makes one more forlorn effort: what shall she do if she really *can't face up to herself? The response that she gets tells her that she cannot remain attached, and, more, that the important person has full confidence in her ability to grow up and away from him. Slowly incorporating a good object in the course of treatment, she makes one more attempt to remain attached and retain thereby both the good and the bad objects. She is denied permission to retain the bad and is given per-*

mission to take the good with her; she responds with pleasure in feeling and accepting the faith of the therapist in her.

My activity speaks for itself. Suggestion, abreaction, manipulation (in the sense of helping her to learn from experience), clarification and interpretation are actively employed in facilitating termination. She is educated to the fact that it is human to have certain feelings and that it is human to employ unwittingly certain maneuvers to avoid mental pain. She is told of future possibilities for feelings of anger and of sadness. It should be noted, however, that every one of these therapeutic devices is attached to the data already obtained from the patient over the course of treatment, as well as to the experiences of the patient and her feelings about them within the treatment.

What I have done here is to emphasize the activity that is necessary to help the patient ' ike the separation. All that has gone before is repeated in capsule form, and I add permission for the patient to feel and to recognize the angry and loving feelings which she has and will have after treatment. This allows for the incorporation of an object that is experienced less ambivalently and with it the freedom to move away from me with less guilt. This then becomes the prerequisite for further growth as an independent adult—growth that she will demonstrate in the follow-up interviews.

Follow-up Interview Five Months after Termination

The patient had had no knowledge that I intended to see her again. My secretary called her and asked if she could come in to see me on a particular date, explaining that my intent was to learn from her how she was getting along. The patient agreed to come.

Dr.: Tell me about you.

Pt.: There isn't too much to tell. I have been pretty good. I have been doing good.

Dr.: Are you nervous about coming here?

Pt.: No. Just a little tired after chasing off to the dentist this morning. I had a busy day. I didn't mind coming. It was rather a surprise when I got the telephone call. On that day I said to my husband that I haven't felt this good in a long time, and then I got the phone call. He said it must be something that you felt that you got the call. I have been doing very well.

Dr.: I want to know how things have been going with you since I last saw you.

Pt.: Well, let's see. Physically, I have been pretty good. My arthritis has been bothering me, but I manage to put up with that. The children have been very good lately. Whether they sense things or not, I don't know. Maybe I have changed, too.

Dr.: Are you going out?

Pt.: Maybe a little too much—too many parties and maybe a little too much else.

Dr.: Do you go out alone?

Pt.: I do if I have to. I just don't go out much with my husband. I mean, I take the children out, I go shopping—I do my own shopping now—I do all my own work because my children each have a part-time job. Instead of me getting a job, they got part-time jobs for spending money, and I take care of the house, which I don't mind. I find it, I don't know, it's a new experience.

Dr.: What is?

Pt.: Well, doing the things that I am doing now and feeling the way I feel. The past few years I hadn't felt this good, wasn't able to do things I wanted to do. But I manage now. I still find days, you know, that I don't feel too secure. Then I find that I just have to put up with it. I don't have anybody to fall back on so I just manage.

Dr.: Fall back on yourself.

Pt.: Right. I just sit and argue with myself instead of picking up the phone and bothering anybody. I fight it out.

Dr.: And how does that work out?

Pt.: I get tired of listening to myself, so I can imagine how everybody else was tired of listening. My husband said I progressed an awful lot.

Dr.: How about your mother?

Pt.: She is still fine. I call her now and then. I am not as faithful as I used to be. About three months ago I told her that I couldn't be chasing down for her all the time, and she, dying all over the place, picked herself up and started to use cabs.

Dr.: Very good.

Pt.: There has been a lot going on from one week to another. It seems like I have something to look forward to all the time now, and I used to—well, I used to hate to see anything coming up because I didn't want to go. Now I am waiting to see what is coming up next week so I can go. I have gone back to going to Mass on Sundays. I am able to go to church, which I haven't done for about a year. So all in all I think I have accomplished quite a bit.

Dr.: It certainly sounds that way.

Pt.: But I still get a little leery. I have my days. But I figure that I just don't want to go out, or I don't want to get on a bus, but the next day I try and push myself and get over it.

Dr.: Do you have any trouble sleeping?

Pt.: No, I sleep well.

Dr.: Do you remember that you had talked about the possibility of getting a job?

Pt.: Like I said, my children put me out of that job . . . So I said I will stay put as long as they are happy and stay with the little ones. That's my job for the summer. When my daughter comes home in early evening, she takes over, and my husband and I go out. We have been going out two or three nights a week, visiting, or for a walk. Tomorrow night we are going out for dinner.

Dr.: Go to the movies?

Pt.: No. That's the next thing to come. It must be two years since I've been in a theater. I have been to drive-ins. My husband would like to go, so I am getting game to give it a try.

Dr.: Do you think that you might be nervous no matter what the picture is?

Pt.: No, probably just the fact of being with a lot of people. I have gone to Mass, and I have gone to parties where there are lots of people, so maybe it won't bother me to go to the movies. Of course, I don't care to see a gruesome movie. I would like to see a comedy.

Dr.: That's why I asked whether it was any kind of movie that you might be nervous about. If that's the only thing you can't do, then you are doing all right, that's not too bad.

Pt.: I can watch television. I like the feeling of being able to go shopping.

Dr.: What about the palpitations?

Pt.: I don't have that any more. I don't have too much of that anxiety. When the children go to the beach, I let them go, but I feel a little anxious. But then I find something to keep me busy.

Dr.: You restrain yourself.

Pt.: I don't say anything any more. I just let them go. I tell them so long, and they come home.

Dr.: You tell me lots of good things that are happening. Now what about the bad things?

Pt.: I don't know of any.

Dr.: Are you quite contented?

Pt.: Everything seems to be going my way. My son got promoted with a good report card, my husband graduated. And that was another thing—I went to his graduation, which I think I have been worrying about for four years, sitting there with all the people. I handled that all right.

Dr.: Have you had any hives?

Pt.: No. I do break out like this around the wrist and the fingers, that's all. They seem to be like water blisters, and then they go away.

Dr.: Are you taking any kind of medication?

Pt.: No. Only Excedrin for headaches.

Dr.: How about your psoriasis?

Pt.: I have that. That doesn't bother me. I have had that for so long, and it doesn't seem to get any worse.

Dr.: Do you remember that, when the last time I saw you, you were quite concerned as to whether you would be able to manage?

Pt.: Make a go of it? I think that I have.

Dr.: It certainly sounds that way.

Pt.: I remember you mentioning that I would want to be able to get in touch with you. I had one such day. I don't know what turned up, I can't recall. I remember saying to my husband if I could get hold of him I would probably call. He asked me if I wanted him to get hold of you, and I said, "No, never mind, I have to take care of the situation myself." That was more at the beginning.

Dr.: Have you missed me? . . .

Pt.: Have I missed coming here to see you? No, I often wonder how you are.

Dr.: That's what I mean.

Pt.: No. I mean, medically no. Personally, yes, I miss you. There will be times during the day when I will say, "I wonder how Dr. Mann is." I talk about the hospital a lot, and if conversation comes up I mention it. I was wondering if you were still here.

Dr.: I am still alive.

Pt.: That comes into everybody's mind. I wonder who is here and who is gone and how they are. It seems funny, but I had said, what if anything really happens and I had to go back and you weren't there—who would I go to? I suppose I would find help here somewhere. Thank God, everything has been progressing.

Dr.: Do you remember, too, that you told me that you would find yourself going to the phone to call somebody. Do you remember who it was?

Pt.: No.

Dr.: Then you might remember that you can't call him.

Pt.: Oh, my father. I don't find myself thinking that way any more. I have tried to push him out of my mind. Like I said to my husband, maybe I ought to leave him alone, maybe he doesn't want me pulling him back. I haven't really put my mind to any dead people, which isn't like me. There were three deaths in my family, and I didn't even go. They wanted to know why. I said, "I care to think of them the way they were," and I just didn't go. I was criticized, but I didn't care.

Dr.: Are you better able to say no?

Pt.: I learned and I practiced to say no. There have been several things, and I just didn't bother. The only time I put myself out and say yes is when my husband asks me to go some place. I push myself and go for his sake.

Dr.: I remember that when I last saw you you were quite eager to get pregnant.

Pt.: Not so now.

Dr.: No?

Pt.: I think I have enough to handle for now. I think maybe that was an out. Like I said to my husband, maybe if I got pregnant and got back into the hospital—but I think I can stay put and take care of what I have.

Dr.: You do recognize that that was a way out, to be pregnant, go into the hospital, and be taken care of?

Pt.: I think I had that on my mind because I hadn't felt so good until I had my last baby and I was in the hospital, and it seemed like a miracle that I felt so good. But I found out that I can get by on my own without going back. I don't think that I will look for any more trouble than I already have. I don't know if my husband spoke to the children or what happened—they all seemed to have turned over new leafs.

Dr.: Tell me about the worrying about all the terrible things that you are afraid will happen to them.

Pt.: I don't seem to worry as much about that now. When they go out, I figure if it is going to happen, it's going to happen whether I worry or not, and worrying isn't going to stop it.

Dr.: Of course. That's true.

Pt.: There is nothing much I can do about it except just go on about my business and let things go. It has been working out so far. So I think that I have progressed a lot.

Dr.: I do, too. I will have to give you an A.

Pt.: A in effort.

Dr.: A gold star on your report card.

Pt.: That's what my son was saying yesterday. He deserves an A. He is getting a bicycle for that, so maybe I ought to get a car. I'll have to tell my husband about that.

Dr.: I think that you should be very much pleased with that.

Pt.: Oh, I am.

Dr.: With what you are doing and how much you have been able to do on your own.

Pt.: Just going out is the pleasure right there, going out and enjoying myself.

Dr.: I want to thank you very much for coming in.

Pt.: I thank you for asking me to come in. I thought you had forgotten all about me.

Dr.: Well, you see that you haven't been forgotten.

Pt.: It's nice to know that I am remembered. You don't think—you won't want me to come back again?

Dr.: Do you have to come back again?

Pt.: No, but I didn't think I would be coming back this time.

Dr.: I only asked you to come back to see how you were . . . It was very nice to see you.

Pt.: Very good to see you, Doctor.

Dr.: I am sure that you will go right on—

Pt.: I hope so. I hope you enjoy the summer.

Follow-up Interview One and One-Half Years After Termination

In order not to arouse the expectations of the patient that a second visit with me could well suggest a continuing relationship with me, I asked one of our social workers who had watched the course of treatment over the closed-circuit television to see the patient for me. The particular social worker was skilled and sensitive in her work, so that I felt confident in her appraisal of the patient. Interestingly, when the social worker called to make an appointment with the patient, the patient said it would be difficult for her to arrange a babysitter, whereupon she quickly accepted the social worker's offer of a home visit.

The children all seemed to be getting along quite well. Daughter Jessica continued to be the worrying and complaining child previously described by the patient as being like herself. The patient hoped that this child would not need psychiatric help, and showed recognition of her impulse to place Jessica in the same position she had been in at the same age by remarking that she tries not to ask Jessica to help too much and makes herself remember that Jessica needs time to play outside the home.

The patient said that she has enjoyed being with her husband more in the last year than for many years previously. He is more relaxed now that she can sleep all night without waking him. They go out together, but she often goes out alone shopping or for a walk. She does not take any medication and feels that an occasional drink does her more good than pills. She has no head pains and no longer wakes up at night afraid she will die. She has taken off about twenty pounds, and she feels more relaxed with her children, her husband, and her mother.

She said that one of the things she realized in talking with Dr. Mann was that she used to be afraid to disagree with her mother and later would feel very resentful. She has been able to say no to her mother and is able to stand up for her children when mother disapproves of their behavior or dress. The patient has encouraged her mother to develop some friendships with women her own age, so that now when the patient calls her mother, the mother is often out with friends.

She often thinks about Dr. Mann and her visits to the hospital, feeling thankful that she went. She regrets that she did not go much earlier, because she feels that ten years of her life were wasted. She felt that she could talk to Dr. Mann, although the first few minutes had been hard each time because she did not know where to start. She added that he always wanted to hear what was on her mind. The social worker asked whether she thought she would call Dr. Mann again if she ever needed further help. She said she hoped she would not have to; moreover, she did not know if she would be able to reach Dr. Mann because he is very busy, but she thought that someone would be able to talk to her. The patient asked the social worker to give her greetings to Dr. Mann.

Index

Abreaction, as therapeutic technique, 49, 53

Activity-passivity conflict, 25–28

Adolescence: concept of time during, 5–6; suitability of time-limited psychotherapy for patients in, 76–77

Agreement, *see* Treatment agreement

Alcoholism, 73–74

Alexander, F., 13, 46, 50

Alpert, R., 6

Anamnesis, associative, 19–20, 22

Anger, 75

Anti-intellectualism, prevalence of, 47

Bellak, L., 13–14

Bergler, E., 21

Bibring, E., 49–50, 54

Bonaparte, Marie, 5–6

Borderline syndrome, 74–75, 76

Bram, Mrs. Paula, 24n

Brief psychotherapy, 30; defined, 13–14

Buddha, Third Noble Truth of, 6–7

Central issue, 17–20, 23, 34, 81–82

Childhood, "paradise" of, 5

Clarification, use of, as therapeutic technique, 50, 52–53, 56, 58

Conflict situations, types of, 25–29

Dass, Baba Ram, 6–7

Daydreams, and sense of time, 6

Defenses, 17, 19

Dependence, on the therapist, 58

Depression, 72, 75

Depressive position, 7–8, 24

Deutsch, Felix, 19–20

Diagnosis, in time-limited psychotherapy, 73–75

Dreams, and sense of time, 6

Drugs, and sense of time, 6

Dying patient, and the concept of time, 8

Education, therapist as transmitter of, 54, 58

Ego: and the sense of time, 7; dysfunction of, in borderline syndrome, 75

Eissler, K., 8

Encounter groups, 47, 53

Father Time, 4

Fisher, R. L., 4

Fisher, S., 4

Fleck, S., 15

Follow-up procedures, 45–46, 70–71

Frank, J., 14, 48

Free association, 19

Freud, Sigmund, 5, 47

Grief, unresolved or delayed, 25–28

Grinker, R. R., 74–75

Heroin, and sense of time, 6

Homosexuality, 73–74

Immortality (limitless time), portrayed as a woman, 4

Independence-dependence conflict, 25–28

Interpretation, as therapeutic technique, 50, 52–53, 56, 58, 60

Intoxication (from drink or drugs), and sense of time, 6

Johnston, M. S. H., 30

Kernberg, O., 74

Leary, Timothy, 6
Love, intoxication of, and sense of
time, 6

Mahler, Margaret, 24
Malan, D. H., 30, 31
Manipulation, as therapeutic technique,
49–50, 54
Marijuana, and sense of time, 6
Maturational crisis, and time-limited
psychotherapy, 76–77
McNair, D. M., 77
Medication, 51
Methodology, lack of, in short-term
therapies, 12–13
Meyer, E., 14–15
Model neurosis, 24–25
Mystic ecstasy, and sense of time, 6

Oberman, Edna, 31
Optimism, of therapist, 51

Parental figures, and perception of
time, 4
Philips, E. L., 30
Plateau in improvement, 55–57
Pleasure principle, 6
Processes, therapeutic, 50
Proskauer, S., 31
Psychoanalysis, for the therapist, 60
Psychotherapy: and the concept of
time, 9–11; five basic techniques
applicable to, 49–50

Rank, Otto, 9–10
Readjustment, therapeutic process of,
50–51
Regression, 32–33
Relationship of patient and therapist,
14, 32, 52, 53–54
Reorientation, therapeutic process of,
50–51

Resistance, to new treatment methods,
78–80
Roheim, G., 21

St. Augustine, 3
Schecter, D. E., 3–4
Schizophrenia, treatment for, 72
Scott, W. Clifford M., 5
Self-esteem: emphasis on patient's, 21,
53; adequate versus diminished or
loss of, 25–27
Self-identity, 75
Semrad, E. V., 13
Separation-individuation crisis, 24–26,
28, 75, 76, 79
Sifneos, P. E., 13, 75
Small, L., 13–14
Stammering, 40, 44
Stereotype, of the analyst or therapist,
48, 53
Structure, of treatment experience, 30
Suggestion: as therapeutic technique,
49; optimism of therapist as form
of, 51
Swartz, Jacob, 76

Termination of psychotherapy: prob-
lem of, 31, 83; reaction of patients
to, 35–38, 58–60
Therapist, and new treatment
methods, 79–80
Transference, 83; cures, 33, 33n
Treatment agreement, 21–23, 32, 81
Treatment, choice of, 72–73
Treatment process, 15–20
Twelve treatment sessions: choice of,
15, 16, 20–21; summaries of, 38–45,
61–71

Uniqueness, of each patient, 29

Weisman, A. D., 3, 8
Winnicott, D. W., 7–8, 24
Wolberg, L. R., 12–13
Wolfe, Thomas, 3